MIDWIFERY PR

Edited by
Jo Alexander, Valerie Levy
and Sarah Roch

' Series: Jo Alexander, Valerie Levy & Sarah Roch 1990

' This Volume: Preconception care — the embryo of health promotion, Joyce Shorney; The organisation of midwifery care, Rosemary Currell; The antenatal booking interview, Rosemary C. Methven; Antenatal preperation of the breasts for breastfeeding, Jo Alexander; Maternal alcohol and tobacco use during pregnancy, Moira Plant; Antenatal Education, Tricia Murphy-Black; Ultrasound — the midwife s role, Jean Proud; The psychology of pregnancy, Joyce Prince and Margaret Adams; Multiple births — parents anxieties and the realities, Jane Spillman

First published 1990 by
THE MACMILLAN PRESS LTD
Houndmills, Basingstoke, Hampshire RG21 2XS
and London
Companies and representatives
throughout the world

ISBN 0–333–53861–7 hardcover
ISBN 0–333–51369–X paperback

A catalogue record for this book is available
from the British Library.

Printed in Hong Kong

Reprinted 1991 (twice), 1992

Acknowledgements

The editors and the publishers wish to thank the following who have kindly given permission for the use of copyright material: Alan R. Liss Inc. for Figure 5.2, Percent Occurance of Abnormalities, Teratology , The Scottish Health Education Group for Figure 5.1, Units of Alcohol .

Every effort has been made to trace all the copyright holders but if any have been inadvertently overlooked the publishers will be pleased to make the necessary arrangements at the first opportunity.

Contents

Other volumes in the Midwifery Practice series

■ **Intrapartum care**   ISBN 0–333–51370–3 (paperback)
                          ISBN 0–333–53862–5 (hardcover)

1. *Rona Campbell*: The place of confinement
2. *Sheila Drayton*: Midwifery care in the first stage of labour
3. *Christine Henderson*: Artificial rupture of the membranes
4. *Judith Grant*: Nutrition and hydration in labour
5. *Alison M. Heywood and Elaine Ho*: Pain relief in midwifery
6. *Jennifer Sleep*: Spontaneous delivery
7. *Valerie Levy*: The midwife's management of the third stage of labour
8. *Carolyn Roth and Janette Brierley*: HIV infection – a midwifery perspective

■ **Postnatal care**   ISBN 0–333–51371–1 (paperback)
                        ISBN 0–333–53863–3 (hardcover)

1. *Jennifer Sleep*: Postnatal perineal care
2. *Sally Inch*: Postnatal care of the breastfeeding mother
3. *Jenifer M. Holden*: Emotional problems following childbirth
4. *Ellena Salariya*: Parental-infant attachment
5. *Janet Rush*: Care of the umbilical cord
6. *Chris Whitby*: Transitional care
7. *Margaret Adams and Joyce Prince*: Care of the grieving parent, with special reference to stillbirth
8. *Rowan Nunnerley*: Quality assurance in postnatal care
9. *Marianne J. G. Mills*: Teenage mothers

Contributors to this volume

Margaret E Adams MSc SRN SCM MTD DN
Queen Charlotte's College of Health Care Studies, Faculty of Midwifery and Women's Health, London.
As an experienced midwife teacher, Margaret Adams' interests are wide, but in particular, she regards the development of interpersonal skills as a priority for midwives. She has written on midwives' styles of communication in the second stage of labour as part of a master's degree in social research methods.

Jo Alexander RN RM MTD PhD JBCNS course 900 (family planning)
Midwifery Education Department, Princess Anne Hospital, Southampton.
Jo Alexander is a Series Editor and details about her are given on the back cover of this book.

Rosemary Currell MPhil BA SRN SCM
Rosie Maternity Hospital, Cambridge.
Rosemary Currell now researches into the functions and information needs of maternity care. Before this she was sister in the antenatal clinic at the West Suffolk Hospital. The concept of continuity of care is one of her particular research interests.

Rosemary C Methven MSc SRN SCM MTD DN (Part A) FETC DANS RCNT
Senior Midwifery Tutor, Post-Basic Studies, Leeds General Infirmary.
Rosemary Methven undertook the research which forms the basis of 'The antenatal booking interview' in part-fulfilment of an MSc in nursing at the University of Manchester.

Tricia Murphy-Black RM RGN RCNT MSc PhD
Nursing Research Unit, University of Edinburgh.
Involved in research since 1977, Tricia Murphy-Black's most recent project concerned postnatal care at home. She was elected Chairman of the Royal College of Midwives UK Council in 1989 and is a member of the National Board for Scotland.

Moira Plant RGN RMN PhD
Research Fellow, Alcohol Research Group, University of Edinburgh.
As well as being a Research Fellow, Moira Plant is temporary advisor to the World Health Organisation and consultant to the European Community's group on drinking and pregnancy. Her publications include the book *Women, Drinking and Pregnancy.*

Joyce Prince BA BSc PhD SRN SCM
Formerly Honorary Lecturer in Psychology, Institute of Obstetrics and Gynaecology, University of London.
Joyce Prince worked as a nurse and midwife before transferring to higher education to read social sciences. Until her recent retirement she was a Research Manager with the DHSS concerned mainly with nursing and midwifery research. She has published on health and social issues.

Jean Proud SRN SCM MTD
Peterborough Maternity Unit.
Jean Proud is sister in charge of obstetric ultrasound and a part-time midwifery tutor. She has worked in ultrasound and pre-natal diagnosis for 11 years and researched into the appearance of the placenta on ultrasound, and an evaluation of its significance as a test of fetal wellbeing.

Joyce Shorney RGN RM RCNT MTD DN (London) FP Certificate
Head of Midwifery Education, Devonshire College of Nursing & Midwifery, Royal Devon & Exeter Hospital, Exeter.
Joyce Shorney is Head of Department of Midwifery Education, an ENB examiner and a member of the Royal College of Midwives. She is also a member of the RCM English Board, the Education Advisory Group, the South West Education Group and she is Regional Representative for the South Western Region. Her research interest is in the reduction of perinatal mortality and morbidity by promoting preconception care.

Jane Spillman MSc SRN SCM
Honorary Research Consultant, Twins & Multiple Births Association, (TAMBA).
Jane Spillman, previously in charge of the Neonatal Unit at Bedford Hospital, is currently studying neonatal needs and provisions for families with twins, triplets and higher multiples. She writes articles and lectures on research and multiple pregnancy, and has delivered papers at a number of international conferences.

Foreword

We must discover the laws on which our profession rests and not invent them.

Anon

In recent years there has been a tremendous shift in approach to antenatal care by midwives.

Women have wanted to be more in control of their own health and progression through pregnancy, and have desired to be more informed in preparing for childbirth. Midwives have tried to respond to the needs of pregnant women by providing a more holistic family-centred approach to care in an ever-changing health care environment.

This first book in the maternity practice series encourages readers to continue to be reflective about their own practice and to challenge traditional practices in midwifery. The authors have provided the latest information on the technical and scientific aspects of antenatal care and the reader is invited to explore further the physical, emotional and practical needs of women.

This series is timely, as the public will increasingly require, and indeed demand, quality care tested through research.

Although midwifery research is relatively new, its growth in recent years has been rapid, and its impact on practice profound. The authors contributing to this series have themselves been instigators of that development through their own research. The aim of this series is to demonstrate and encourage the integration of research and practice. The authors have explored the available sources of knowledge on their own particular subjects and they have provided an excellent guide to the literature, which is both focused on and complimentary to antenatal care.

The student of midwifery will find rich sources of knowledge within this text, and the presentation of the work provides a useful model from which to learn.

Valerie Tickner
Royal College of Midwives Trust

Preface

There is no doubt that the theory underpinning midwifery practice cannot be carved in tablets of stone but must be dynamic and change as new information becomes available. Despite this, it is really only in the last 30 years that research has begun to have any impact on midwifery practice and even now relevant information is not always easily available to practitioners. The Midwives Information and Resource Service (MIDIRS) and the 'Research and the Midwife' conferences have made an outstanding contribution but standard textbooks are often sparsely referenced and full length research papers are time consuming to read.

This three volume series is intended to help to fill the vacuum which exists between the current state of research and the literature readily available and accessible to practitioners. The series offers midwives and senior student midwives a broad-ranging survey and analysis of the research literature relating to the major areas of clinical practice. We hope that it will also prove stimulating to childbearing women, their families and others involved with the maternity care services. The books do not pretend to give the comprehensive coverage of a definitive textbook and indeed their strength derives from the in-depth treatment of a selection of topics. The topic areas were chosen with great care and authors were approached who have a particular research interest and expertise. On the basis of their critical appraisal of the literature the authors make recommendations for clinical practice, and thus the predominant feature of these books is the link made between research and key areas of practice.

The chapters have a common structure which is described below. It is hoped that this will be attractive to readers and assist those reviewing existing policies or wishing to study a topic in still greater depth. Some knowledge of basic research terminology will prove useful, but its lack should not discourage readers.

We owe a debt of gratitude to many people: most of all to our authors who have worked so painstakingly to produce their contributions and many of whom have helped us in numerous other ways; to Sarah Robinson for her early encouragement and to our publishers during the development of the series; and, not least, to all those practitioners and students who made valuable comments on draft material.

We hope that many practitioners will use the books to increase their knowledge, stimulate their interest in research and improve and extend their own practice of the art and science of midwifery.

JA
VL
SR

■ Common structure of chapters

In fulfilment of the aims of the series, each chapter follows a common structure:

1. The introduction offers a digest of the contents;

2. *'It is assumed that you are already aware of the following ...'* establishes the prerequisite knowledge and experience assumed of the reader;

3. The main body of the chapter reviews and analyses the most appropriate and important research literature currently available;

4. The *'Recommendations for clinical practice'* offers suggestions for sound clinical practice based on the author's interpretation of the literature;

5. The *'Practice check'* enables professionals to examine their own practice and the principles and policies influencing their work;

6. Bibliographic sources are covered under *References* (to research) and *Suggestions for further reading.*

■ Further reading on research

The titles listed below are suggested for those who wish to further their knowledge and understanding of research principles.

Cormack D F S (ed) 1984 The Research Process in Nursing. Blackwell Scientific Publications, Oxford
Hockey L 1985 Nursing Research – Mistakes and Misconceptions. Churchill Livingstone, Edinburgh
Tornquist E M 1986 From proposal to publication: an informal guide to writing about nursing research. Addison Wesley, Reading (Massachusetts)

Chapter 1

Preconception care – the embryo of health promotion

Joyce Shorney

Preconception care or preparing for pregnancy is not a new phenomenon and should be considered as an essential part of health promotion. If human life is conceived in the best possible environment this can only assist in reducing perinatal, neonatal and maternal mortality and morbidity thus improving the potential good health of future generations.

One of the earliest references to preconception care is in the Old Testament (*Book of Judges*, Chapter 13):

> An angel of God appeared to the wife of Manoah and said, you are
> barren and have no child but from now on take great care, take
> no wine or strong drink and eat nothing unclean for you will
> conceive and bare a son.

The child born to Manoah was Samson, renowned for his strength and stamina.

For many years advances have been made in obstetric and midwifery care both during the prenatal, intrapartum, postnatal and neonatal periods. These advances include the introduction of better training for doctors and midwives, the selective use of technology, the active management of labour, and the development of neonatal units that provide intensive, high dependency, special and transitional care. Very little attention has been paid, however, to the importance of health prior to and around the time of conception.

Preconception care can be described as common sense health promotion: the concept is to heighten the awareness of the public to the importance of maximum health prior to conception, at the time of fertilisation and during the period of embryonic development. Such an approach can only reduce the incidence of congenital malformations, the birth of preterm and growth retarded babies and birth hypoxia – the four most common causes of perinatal mortality and morbidity.

1

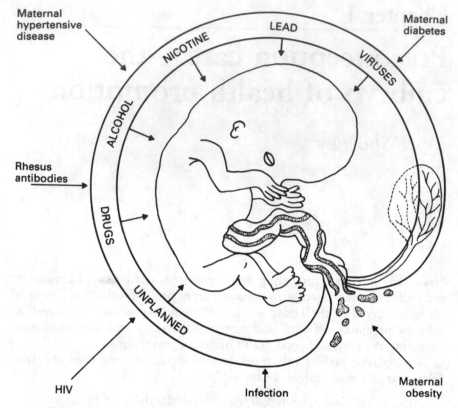

Figure 1.1 Factors adversely affecting fetal growth and development

The aim of this chapter is to demonstrate how health professionals can motivate and assist the parents of the future to prepare both physically and mentally for the miracle of conception – the beginning of a new life.

■ It is assumed that you are already aware of the following:

- The physiology of the menstrual cycle, including hormonal control, phases and possible variations, in order to assist women with awareness of their own fertility;

- The process of spermatogenesis, the production of spermatozoa, their transport to the seminal vesicles and the contents of a normal sample of ejaculate of semen;

- The process of conception and early cell division including the formation of the blastocyst;

● Embryonic and fetal development, including the adverse factors that may interfere with normal cell differentiation.

■ Preconception care: a critical appraisal

Preconception care is a phenomenon of the last decade and although many articles have been written about the importance of health prior to conception very little validated research has been published recently. However, when providing preconception care the following research literature should be considered.

☐ Nutrition

In 1945 Dr Weston Price stated that the refined and valueless diet of modern man had disastrous consequences for fetal integrity. Having travelled the globe, he also found that people eating natural foods, regardless of their country of origin, produced children with fewer congenital disadvantages.

Dr Frank Pottenger's animal experiments proved that dietary manipulation could reduce the incidence of disorders previously thought to be genetic in origin (Pottenger 1983). In Holland, the 'Hunger Winter' (October 1944 to May 1945) demonstrated that babies conceived during the worst food shortage resulted in a perinatal mortality of 65 per 1000 (30–40 per 1000 being the normal range). A study of this was published by Stein *et al* in 1975 and by Wynn and Wynn (1981).

It is also known that many specialised body cells, for example, lymphocytes, take months to recover from deficiencies in essential nutrients so couples must be counselled on the importance of good nutrition prior to conception as well as during pregnancy (Chamberlain & Lumley 1986). Delayed effects of the Dutch Hunger Winter included, for example, a greatly increased incidence of congenital malformation and embryonic growth retardation (Stein *et al* 1975; Wynn & Wynn 1981).

Dietary deficiency is also associated with early spontaneous abortion (Ebbs *et al* 1941; Laurence *et al* 1980).

Smithells *et al* (1980) reported apparent reductions in neural tube defects in babies whose mothers had been given periconceptual vitamin supplementation; they also found that such supplements had a similar effect on the incidence of cleft lip and palate. The periconceptual administration of multivitamins has now been investigated further and concern expressed relating to the massive doses of nonspecific pharmacological agents with unknown side effects. In 1986 the Medical Research Council and the Royal College of Obstetricians and Gynaecologists mounted a multi-centred, randomised trial to examine the problems of vitamins and folate in the

4 · Antenatal Care

pregnancy period, the results of which have not yet been published. An article in the *British Medical Journal* by Professor Rodney Harris (1988) discusses some of the controversial issues relating to this randomised double-blind trial that is examining the efficacy of the different ingredients of Pregnavite Forte F in women who have had a fetus with a neural tube defect.

A number of studies carried out in the USA over the last 2 decades (Oberleas *et al* 1972; Williams 1973; Pfeiffer 1975, 1978; Ward 1987) demonstrate that a deficiency in zinc and manganese can affect the fetus adversely and that modern diet has been shown to be deficient in these elements. Research has also indicated that atmospheric pollution may interfere with the metabolism of certain minerals as may deficiencies in vitamins and essential amino acids (Roels *et al* 1978; Ward 1987). Other factors that may deplete the body of essential vitamins and trace elements are the oral contraceptive pill (Larsson-Cohn 1975; Grant 1985), copper piping in soft water areas (Elkington 1985) and alcohol consumption leading to congenital abnormality and intrauterine growth retardation (Hansen *et al* 1978; Plant 1987).

□ Weight and height

The Quetelet Index (normal range 20–5) can be used to assess the required weight for height before the woman contemplates pregnancy. This is calculated as follows:

$$\frac{\text{WEIGHT IN KILOGRAMS}}{\text{HEIGHT IN METRES}^2}$$

For example:

$$\frac{58.5\,\text{kg}}{1.62 \times 1.62} = 22.3$$

An index of less than 20 indicates that the woman is underweight suggesting long term health hazards and emotional tenseness. Both of these factors may lead to subfertility and, during pregnancy, to placental dysfunction and associated intrauterine growth retardation. An index of over 30 indicates obesity which increases pregnancy risks by contributing to hypertensive disease and thrombo-embolic complications. From a practical point of view, obesity makes clinical assessment of uterine growth and fetal presentation very difficult.

□ Genetic counselling

Prepregnancy genetic counselling, which includes obtaining a detailed family history and the taking of blood for chromosome analysis from both partners, will enable the counsellor to predict the risk factors and give any appropriate preconception advice. Details of prenatal screening can also be discussed such as chorionic villus sampling, fetoscopy, amniocentesis and ultrasonography that detect abnormality and, if present, a termination of pregnancy can be offered under Clause 4 of the Abortion Act 1967.

■ Pre-existing medical disorders

Existing medical disorders may either be adversely affected by the pregnancy or increase the risk of pregnancy to both the woman and the fetus. It is therefore important that women with certain disorders should obtain preconception counselling in order to minimise these risks.

□ Hypertension

Hypertension predisposes to superimposed pre-eclampsia (Butler & Bonham 1963). If a woman suffers from hypertension before conception, therefore, the condition should be fully investigated and, if necessary, controlled with medication.

The latest *Confidential Enquiries into Maternal Mortality in England and Wales 1982–1984* (Department of Health 1989) reports that hypertensive disease is one of the two most common causes of maternal death (the other being pulmonary embolism). Hypertensive disease is also associated with fetal loss due to placental dysfunction leading to intrauterine growth retardation and an increased incidence of preterm delivery. It is therefore important to investigate and control hypertensive disease prior to pregnancy.

□ Diabetes Mellitus

Pregnancy is often described as diabetogenic, and clinical studies have demonstrated that the diabetic state becomes less stable in pregnancy and requires careful monitoring with blood glucose levels (Drury 1985; Gillmer 1985). There is also an associated increase in pre-eclampsia, polyhydramnios, preterm labour, macrosomia leading to shoulder dystocia, congenital abnormality and perinatal death. It is therefore essential to provide a pre-pregnancy counselling service using glycosylated haemoglobin (HbA_1) levels to provide strict diabetic control thus preventing hyperglycaemia around conception which has been shown to interfere with normal organogenesis (especially of the neural tube, heart and kidneys) and to reduce other complications of pregnancy associated with an unstable diabetic state (Burden 1985).

☐ Phenylketonuria

This inborn error of metabolism involving phenylalanine can be treated effectively by a low phenylalanine diet in the affected child. It is recessively inherited (the incidence being one in four if both parents carry the affected autosome) and occurs in 10 000–15 000 pregnancies.

High levels of phenylalanine in pregnancy, which would occur in a woman who was treated as a child for phenylketonuria but has ceased taking her special diet, are associated with abortion, intrauterine growth retardation, congenital heart defect, microcephaly and mental retardation. The reintroduction of a low phenylalanine diet prior to pregnancy has been shown to improve fetal prognosis (Scott *et al* 1980; Davidson *et al* 1981).

☐ Epilepsy

Anticonvulsant therapy, particularly phenytoin, has been shown to be teratogenic and women suffering from epilepsy should be advised to receive medical advice prior to conception (Wood & Bexley 1981).

Further reference to other less common medical disorders and their effect on pregnancy is beyond the scope of this text but has been covered by Chamberlain and Lumley (1986).

■ Social poisons

☐ Tobacco and alcohol

Smoking is a health hazard to both the mother and the fetus. There is abundant evidence in the literature that smoking during pregnancy is a major cause of prenatal complications leading to handicap and deformity in the neonate. As early as 1957, Simpson reported that babies born to women who smoke during pregnancy are 200 grams lighter on average than babies born to non-smoking mothers. This may not in itself be biologically significant but the incidence of prematurity, intrauterine growth retardation, birth hypoxia and sudden infant death syndrome is increased.

The consumption of alcohol around the time of conception and during pregnancy is known to be associated with spontaneous abortion, low birthweight and with fetal alcohol syndrome (Plant 1987). Centuries ago, the Greek philosophers were aware of the dangers of alcohol. Plato's view was that, 'It is not right that procreation should be the work of bodies dissolved by excess wine but rather that the embryo should be compacted firmly, steadily and quietly in the womb' (Laws, b.775c; reissued 1970). Aristotle (cited by Burton 1621) warned that 'foolish, drunken or hare brained women for the most part bring forth children like unto themselves morose and languid'.

For further discussion of this topic, the reader is referred to Chapter 5, 'Maternal alcohol and tobacco use during pregnancy' by Moira Plant.

☐ Drugs

Medication in itself may have teratogenic effects on the developing fetus, although the abnormality may not be directly caused by the drug but may be associated with a drug-nutrient interaction. Dickenson, in 1980, suggested that the drug thalidomide may have interacted with riboflavin as a deficiency of riboflavin in animals produced similar malformations. There is also fairly conclusive evidence that women taking anticonvulsant drugs to control epilepsy are more likely to give birth to a malformed baby and women receiving Vitamin A therapeutically for some skin disorders should cease treatment a year prior to conception because of the teratogenic affects of the high levels of Vitamin A (Gal *et al* 1972). Further detailed information is given by Wood and Bexley (1981).

■ Environmental pollutants

Professor Bryce Smith of the Unversity of Reading has drawn attention to the fact that lead pollution in the atmosphere causes stillbirth, congenital damage to the brain and central nervous system resulting in retardation (Bryce Smith 1980). The use of unleaded petrol should therefore be promoted. Other environmental pollutants are cadmium, mercury, chemical agents such as anaesthetic gases, solvents, pesticides and ionising radiation. Prolonged exposure to visual display units may present another hazard but this requires further research. Pollutants may cause problems such as impotence and menstrual disorders leading to subfertility and, during pregnancy, spontaneous abortion, congenital abnormalities and cancers in the children.

A couple planning to start a family should be advised that employers are obliged by law to inform them of any chemicals or other processes known to be hazardous to the developing embryo within their place of work.

■ Exercise and stress

Regular vigorous exercise as undertaken by highly trained athletes has been shown (Bullard 1981) to be associated with infertility, congenital malformations, preterm labour, premature placental separation, fetal distress, reduced birth weight and difficult labours which are thought to be associated with increased rigidity of the pelvic floor muscles, pelvic joints and ligaments. Emotional stress has been demonstrated to be linked to infertility and pregnancy complications (Nucholls *et al* 1972). The research undertaken on the effects of exercise is very limited and there is insufficient evidence to date to support further recommendations related to the benefits or hazards of exercise in pregnancy on the healthy woman (Chamberlain & Lumley 1986). The complications associated with stress include accidental injury during pregnancy, psychological disorders, perinatal death, postpartum infection and haemorrhage (Laukaran & van den Berg 1980).

■ Family planning

If couples seeking preconception counselling are using either the oral contraceptive pill or the intrauterine contraceptive device, specific advice should be given on the cessation of these methods and the timing of conception.

□ Hormonal methods

Although the combined (oestrogen and progestogen) oral contraceptive pill is an efficient method of contraception, it should be discontinued three to six months prior to conception so that a regular ovulatory and menstrual cycle can be resumed (Bamfield 1989). This increases the accuracy of estimating the expected date of delivery and enables the oestrogen and progesterone levels to return to normal. There is now considerable literature demonstrating that the interaction of contraceptive agents with nutrients and vitamins results in decreased availability of pyridoxine leading to decreased synthesis of serotonin and the decreased absorption of zinc leading to zinc deficiency both of which are teratogenic (Larsson-Cohn 1975; Vessey *et al* 1978).

The combined pill acts as a contraceptive by suppressing ovulation, rendering the cervical mucus hostile to sperm and the endometrium unfavourable for implantation. These physiological changes need to revert to normal for a healthy conception to occur.

The mini (progesterone only) pill may not suppress ovulation but its other actions are similar to the combined pill and should also be discontinued three to six months prior to conception (Bamfield 1989).

□ Intrauterine contraceptive device

The intrauterine contraceptive device (IUCD) is a relatively efficient form of contraception, being 97–8 per cent effective. It is thought that the presence of this device in the uterine cavity prevents implantation and the copper component, if present, reduces the favourability of the endometrium for implantation. A woman using this form of contraception should be advised to wait three to six months following its removal before embarking upon a pregnancy to enable the endometrium to become healthy, vascular and secretory (Bamfield 1989). Copper has also been shown to interfere with the absorption of zinc a trace element which is essential for normal embryonic development (Zipper *et al* 1969). The effects of the copper present on the intrauterine device should therefore be given time to subside before conception.

■ Subfertility

If a couple have been having regular unprotected intercourse for a year without achieving a pregnancy, they are described as 'subfertile'. It is found (Bamfield 1989) that in one third of cases male factors are responsible and these include defective spermatogenesis, abnormality of the seminal ducts and impaired secretions from the seminal vesicles or the prostate gland, one third relate to female factors such as defective ovulation caused by endocrine or ovarian disorders, abnormality or obstruction in the fallopian tube, cervical infection or unfavourable mucus preventing sperm penetration, anti-sperm antibodies, uterine abnormalities or hormonal imbalance preventing implantation. In the remaining third of cases there may be a combination of factors such as defective ovulation and a low sperm count (Bamfield 1989).

An infertile couple is one in whom pregnancy has been proved to be impossible without artificial intervention. Such couples require sympathetic counselling and should receive the best preconception advice.

■ Screening for health

This should be carried out in order to detect any complications that have not previously been identified, but which require advice and/or treatment prior to conception.

□ Urinalysis

The urine should be examined for the presence of abnormal constituents, as listed below.

- *Proteinuria* – having excluded contamination this may indicate pyelonephritis or chronic renal disease, which if untreated debilitates physical health and predisposes to abortion, preterm labour, anaemia, intrauterine growth retardation also thrombo-embolic complications and haemorrhage if anaemia is present. Renal investigations are easier to undertake and interpret in the non-pregnant state.

- *Glycosuria* – this may be due to a high carbohydrate intake, to increased glomerular filtration and a lowered renal threshold, or to diabetes mellitus which requires stabilisation prior to conception (see page 5).

- *Ketonuria* – this indicates dehydration and electrolyte imbalance and may be caused by vomiting and diarrhoea or associated with unstable diabetes mellitus.

☐ **Blood tests**

These should include screening for:

- Rubella antibodies (after which rubella vaccination should be offered to susceptible women, see below);

- Haemoglobin level – as anaemia is best investigated and treated prior to pregnancy;

- Haemoglobinopathies, such as thalassaemia and sickle cell anaemia, which are responsible for significant mortality and morbidity in the mother and fetus/baby (Tuck *et al* 1983; Chamberlain & Lumley 1986);

- Syphilis (screening for sexually transmitted diseases is controversial in the preconception period as the woman is likely to become reinfected prior to conception);

- Screening for HIV antibodies should be offered to women in high risk groups. Pre- and post-test counselling services are essential and the reader is referred to the chapter on 'HIV infection: a midwifery perspective' by Carolyn Roth and Janette Brierley in the volume in this series on *Intrapartum Care*.

☐ **Rubella vaccination**

As the rubella virus crosses the placental barrier and has a teratogenic effect on the fetus it is important that women who are found to be rubella susceptible are offered vaccination. They should be advised to avoid conception for three months and then arrange a further blood test to confirm rubella immunity (Banatvala 1982). In the meantime effective contraceptive advice needs to be given and a hormonal injectable, such as Depo-provera, may be prescribed.

As it has now been demonstrated that rubella vaccination provides immunity for varying periods of time in each individual (Banatvala 1982) women should be advised to have their rubella status checked prior to each pregnancy. Natural rubella immunity provides life long protection.

☐ Ovulatory and menstrual cycle

Women should have an awareness of the physiology of their menstrual cycle and be advised to record the first day of each menstrual period so that when conception occurs, the estimated date of confinement can be more accurately assessed and early prenatal care initiated. It is also important for the woman to be aware of the normal length of her cycle and period of menses.

Having outlined some of the factors that need to be considered before providing preconception care, it is now necessary to consider how the relevant information can be disseminated to couples wishing to start a family.

■ Clinical practice

Preconception care may be visualised as a bridge between the Family Planning Clinic that provides contraception in preparation for a planned conception and the first prenatal visit early in pregnancy. It is a time when women and their partners should be encouraged to do something positive towards preparing for the conception and birth of another very precious human being.

Prepregnancy care can be divided into two specific aspects – health promotion and medical care.

☐ Health promotion

This is part of total education for living and can be provided in the following ways.

● The role of parents – preparation for parenthood should begin in the home where children are brought up in a safe environment ensuring both physical and emotional stability, respect for each other and an awareness of their role in society. Therefore the first aim should be to help parents to prepare their children to be responsible parents themselves. This can be done through radio or television, by using leaflets, or through health professionals attending Parents' Association meetings.

- *Health education in schools* – prepregnancy advice can be provided in schools by including health education, sexuality, reproduction and preparation for responsible parenthood in the curriculum. Health professionals may be invited to contribute to these sessions. A positive portrayal of human sexuality can be fostered in classroom sessions, encouraging the pupils to see it as something special, to be treasured within a loving relationship, and resulting in the conception of a planned and much wanted human being.

- *Family planning clinics* – family planning services have a duty to provide safe and efficient methods of contraception at the same time giving advice relating to a planned and healthy conception. In preconception care the questions relating to contraception are specifically concerned with the timing of conception following the discontinuation of the chosen method of birth control and these should be considered individually at the time of consultation.

- *Well women clinics* – these are provided in many large towns and cities to promote an awareness of health and provide facilities for screening such as breast examination and cervical cytology. These facilities should be further developed to include prepregnancy advice and screening. In some areas 'well men clinics' are also being introduced.

- *Occupational health departments* – facilities should be developed in occupational health departments, particularly in industry, to provide advice and screening prior to conception.

- *Mobile van 'Health for All'* – this is an ideal way of promoting health in a rural community and has recently been introduced within the Exeter Health Authority. Its aims include prepregnancy advice and preparation for parenthood.

- *Health centres* – the promotion of health as well as the treatment of disease is an integral part of the role of the primary health care team; community midwives, GPs, health visitors and other professionals.

- *The media* – it is essential to promote the concept of prepregnancy care in journals, magazines, newspapers, on the radio and television.

- *Phone-in services* – 'Healthline' is a service provided by the Exeter Health Authority that enables the public to telephone a central point and listen to a tape on the health subject of their choice. An advantage of this method is that it can be followed in the privacy of the individual's own home. The tape on preparing for pregnancy gives the midwives' central telephone number which has an answerphone for further information and enables a midwife to visit the couple as required.

☐ Medical care

Medical care is provided in preconception clinics by midwives and doctors and will include physical examinations and laboratory tests. Preconception clinics are now being set up within health centres, general practices and in hospitals to provide specific and specialist advice (Chamberlain 1982; Witchalls 1984).

The organisation 'Foresight' was formed to ensure that all possible steps were taken to enable every baby that is born into this world is as free as possible from congenital deformity and mental damage and is in perfect health. Publications by Foresight include *Guidelines for Future Parents* (Dickerson 1980) and *Planning for a Healthy Baby* (Barnes & Bradley 1990).

When providing preconception care all the aspects covered in the cycle of care shown in Fig. 1.2 should be considered. These include the following.

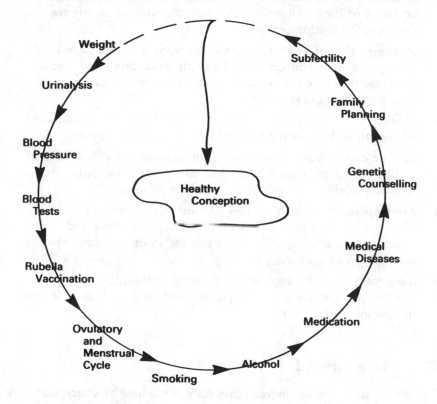

Figure 1.2 The preconception cycle of care

- *Weight* – an appropriate weight in relation to height suggests good health and the Quetelet formula can be used to calculate this (see page 4). Dietary advice should be given and women who are excessively overweight or underweight should be referred to a dietitian.

- *Urinalysis* – a midstream specimen of urine should be obtained and tested for abnormal constituents. Any deviation from the normal should be referred for further investigation.

- *Blood pressure* – the diastolic blood pressure should not exceed 80–85mmHg in the reproductive years, the systolic blood pressure may vary with physical exertion, excitement or stress but will settle with rest. Any hypertension should be referred to a doctor for investigation and if necessary treatment.

- *Blood tests* – blood should be taken to assess rubella status and haemoglobin level as a matter of routine. Rubella vaccination should be offered to all susceptible women before conception or in the postnatal period to provide protection in a subsequent pregnancy. Other specific tests have been described on page 10.

- *Ovulatory and menstrual cycles* – women should be encouraged to be aware of their menstrual cycles and to record accurately the first day of each monthly period.

- *Smoking, alcohol and medication* – the woman should be advised ideally to give up smoking, avoid any alcoholic drink and take no self-prescribed medications as these can all have adverse effects on fetal growth and development.

- *Medical diseases* – women with existing health problems should be advised to seek medical advice before attempting to conceive.

- *Genetic counselling* – if inherited disorders occur in either partner's family, the couple should be referred to a genetic counsellor for specialist advice. Self-referral is possible in many areas.

- *Family planning* – those doctors and nurses working in this field are ideally situated to provide general preconception advice and screening as well as specific advice relating to the cessation of contraceptive methods.

- *Subfertility* – the management of subfertility provides the best possible preconception care by professionals and the highest level of motivation by the couple.

■ Looking forward

The above are the basic prerequisites only for a healthy conception and further research must be undertaken as the advantages of preparing for pregnancy are easy to identify in theory but will take some years to prove in practice. Some examples of the theoretical cost-effectiveness of preconception care are the predicted reduction in:

- The number of prenatal women requiring hospital inpatient care because of pregnancy associated complications – the cost of which is £133 per day (Exeter Health Authority's 1989 figures);

- The reduction in neonates requiring intensive and high dependency care (Exeter Health Authority's 1989 figures estimate the approximate cost of one intensive care cot at £400 a day).

Good health before conception is not an absolute guarantee of the birth of a normal healthy baby, but it is logical to presume that a planned healthy conception will reduce the risk of mortality and morbidity in both mother and baby. There is also statistical evidence (HC 1980, 1984; Sweet 1988) that perinatal mortality in particular occurs more commonly amongst unplanned pregnancies, the lower socio-economic groups, young unsupported women, and those women with pre-existing medical disorders and previous obstetrical complications. A survey into perinatal deaths conducted in Exeter (Brimblecombe *et al* 1984) involved interviewing the parents and arranging a case conference of all health professionals involved, in an effort to identify any underlying causes and to study the support provided to the grieving parents. This has resulted in a greater awareness of the need to provide preconception advice but in many cases no identifiable cause was found. It is therefore important that health professionals and particularly the midwife explore all the avenues open to them in the provision of prepregnancy care. This will require dedication and perseverance as attitudes and practices need to change in both the public and the professionals.

It is important to promote good health in the widest possible context, both physical and psychological, to enable conception to occur in optimum conditions. Over the last decade, interest in prepregnancy care has increased considerably but much research is still required to demonstrate that a healthy conception does indeed reduce prenatal complications as well as perinatal, neonatal and maternal morbidity and mortality.

■ Practice check

- What facilities are at present offered in the area in which you work to provide preconception advice?

- Does your Health Promotion Department have leaflets, slides or videos on the importance of health prior to conception?

- Are health professionals involved in the local school curriculum on preparing for healthy parenthood?

- Where are the local family planning facilities provided and are the doctors and nurses aware of the importance of screening for health and giving preconception advice?

- Where is your genetic counsellor located and what is the local system for referral?

- Who is the best person to provide preconception care?

- What acceptable venues are available in which to set up a preconception clinic?

- How can you reach those at greatest risk of pregnancy complications, perinatal, neonatal and maternal mortality and morbidity?

- Are there any 'well persons' clinics' or women's centres in your area?

- Does the health authority have a mobile van to visit public car parks, industry and rural villages to help the public at large become more aware about health issues?

- What facilities for preconception care have been included in your health authority's future strategical plans?

- Have you a local phone-in 'Health Line' that gives advice on a wide variety of health subjects?

- How do your local perinatal, neonatal and maternal mortality statistics compare with previous years and the national average?

- Does your area undertake a confidential enquiry into perinatal death with recommendations for future practice?

- Have you read any articles or books, or attended study sessions on preconception care?

- What are you personally going to do within your present resources and funds available to promote health prior to conception?

■ References

Bamfield T 1989 Preparing for pregnancy. In Bennett V R, Brown L K (eds) Myles textbook for midwives (11th ed). Churchill Livingstone, Edinburgh
Bamphylde H 1984 Countdown to a healthy baby. Collins, London
Banatvala J E 1982 Rubella vaccination – remaining problems. British Medical Journal 284: 1285–86

Barnes B, Bradley S G 1990 Planning for a healthy baby. Foresight, Godalming

Brimblecombe F, Bastow M, Jones J, Kennedy N, Wadsworth J 1984 Enquiries into perinatal and early childhood deaths in a health care district. Archives of Disease in Childhood 59: 682–87

Bryce Smith D 1980 Lead and brain functioning. In Birch G C, Parker K J (eds). Food and Health. Applied Sciences Publishing, London

Bullard J A 1981 Exercise in Pregnancy. Canadian Family Physician 27: 977–82

Burden A C 1985 Diabetic control during pregnancy. Practical Diabetes 2 (5): 16–17

Burton R 1621 Anatomy of melancholy, Vol I(1.2). William Tegg, London

Butler N R, Bonham D G 1963 Perinatal mortality. Livingstone, Edinburgh: 86–100

Chamberlain G 1982 The role of the prepregnancy clinic. Novum 21: 6

Chamberlain G, Lumley J 1986 Prepregnancy care: a manual for practice. John Wiley, Chichester

Crawford M d'A 1985 Papers on preconceptual genetic counselling. First Symposium on Preconception Care Charing Cross Hospital, 4th July 1985: 86

Crosby W H 1977 Fetal malnutrition: an appraisal of correlated factors. American Journal of Obstetrics and Gynecology 128 (1): 22–31

Davidson D C, Isherwood D M, Ireland J T, Page P G, 1981 Outcome of pregnancy in a phenylketonuric mother after low phenylalanine diet introduced from the ninth week of pregnancy. European Journal of Paediatrics 137: 45–8.

Department of Health 1989 Confidential enquiries into maternal deaths in England and Wales 1982–1984. HMSO, London

Dickerson J W T 1980 Guidelines for future parents, environmental factors and foetal health. Foresight, Godalming

Donnai D 1986 Prepregnancy care (Chapter 2): 11. John Wiley, Chichester

Drury M I 1985 Diabetes in pregnancy. Practical Diabetes 2 (5): 3

Ebbs J H, Tisdall O O, Scott W A 1941 The influences of prenatal diet on the mother and child. Journal of Nutrition 22: 515–26

Elkington J 1985 The poisoned womb. Viking, Harmondsworth

Gal I, Sharman I, Pryse-Davies J 1972 Vitamin A in relation to human congenital malformations. Advances in teratology 5: 143

Gillmer M D G 1985 Obstetric management of diabetes. Practical Diabetes 2 (6); 4–5

Grant E 1985 The bitter Pill. Corgi, London

Haddad F 1986 Update on preconception care. Journal of Obstetrics and Gynaecology 6 (Supplement 2): S119–S121

Hansen J W, Streissguth A P, Smith D W 1978 The effects of moderate alcohol consumption on fetal growth and morphogenesis. Journal of Paediatrics 92: 457–60

Harris R 1988 Vitamins and neural tube defects. British Medical Journal 296: 80–1

House of Commons Social Services Committee (HC) 1980 Report on perinatal and neonatal mortality (Short Report). HMSO, London

House of Commons Social Services Committee (HC) 1984 Follow-up report on perinatal and neonatal mortality. HMSO, London

Larsson-Cohn U 1975 Oral contraceptives and vitamins: a review. American Journal of Obstetrics and Gynaecology 121 (i): 84–90

Laukaran V H, van den Berg B J 1980 The relationships of maternal attitude to pregnancy outcomes and obstetric complications. American Journal of Obstetrics and Gynaecology 136: 374–79

Laurence K M, James N, Miller M, Campbell H 1980 Increased risk of reoccurrence of pregnancies complicated by fetal neural tube defects and possible benefit of dietary counselling. British Medical Journal 281: 1592–94

Maternity Alliance Getting fit for pregnancy. Maternity Alliance, London

Mortimer P 1984 Getting fit for a baby (Family Doctor booklet). BMA, London

Mothercare/Royal College of Midwives 1987 Before you conceive. Mothercare Ltd, Watford

National Childbirth Trust Healthy babies begin before you're pregnant. NCT, Leeds

New Era 1980 Hair analysis reveals the secrets of your health. New Era Laboratories, London

Nucholls K B, Casel J, Kaplan B H 1972 Psychosocial assets, life crises and the prognosis of pregnancy. American Journal of Epidemiology 95: 431–44

Oberleas D, Caldwell D, Prasad A 1972 Trace elements and behaviour. International review of neurobiology 85: Supplement

Pfeiffer C C 1975 Mental and elemental nutrients. Keats, New Canaan CT

Pfeiffer C C 1978 Zinc and other micronutrients. Keats, New Canaan CT

Plant M L 1987 Women, drinking and pregnancy. Tavistock Publications, London

Plato Laws. Reissued 1970 as a Penguin Classics edition. Penguin Books, Harmondsworth

Pottenger F M Jnr 1983 Pottenger's cats. Pottenger-Price Nutrition Foundation, La Mesa CA

Price W A 1945 (Reissued 1977) Nutrition and physical degeneration. Price-Pottenger Nutrition Foundation. LA Mesa, California

Read A P, Fielding D W, Walker S, Schorah C J, Wild J (1983) Further experience of vitamin supplementation for prevention of neural tube defect recurrences. Lancet i: 1027–31

Read J M T 1982 Prenatal care – A lesson from Holland. Middle East Health 6 (12): 22–3

Robarts J 1988 Preparing for pregnancy. Faber & Faber, London

Roels H, Humermont G, Butcher J P, Lauverys R 1978 Placental Transfer of lead, mercury, cadmium and carbon monoxide in woman. Environmental Review 16: 236

Scott T M, Morton Fyffe W, McKay Hart D 1980 Maternal phenylketonuria abnormal baby despite low phenylalanine diet during pregnancy. Archives of Diseases in Childhood 55: 634–39

Shorney J M T (1983) Preconception care. Nursing Mirror Midwifery Forum 157(14) Supplement: i–ii

Shorney J M T 1985 Exeter Midwives Advisory Centre. Midwives Chronicle 98(1164): 14–15

Simpson W J A 1957 A preliminary report on cigarette smoking and the incidence of prematurity. American Journal of Obstetrics and Gynecology 73: 808

Smithells R W, Sheppard S, Schorah C J, Seller M J, Nevin N C, Harris R, Read

A P, Fielding D W 1980 Possible prevention of neural tube defects by periconceptual vitamin supplementation. Lancet i: 339–40

Stein Z A, Susser M, Saenger G, Marolla F 1975 Famine and human development: the Dutch Hunger Winter of 1944–1945. Oxford University Press, New York

Sweet B R 1988 Mayes midwifery (11th ed): 571–72. Baillière Tindall, London

Taylor J B 1979 Examine patients for fitness for pregnancy. Journal of the Royal College of General Practitioners 29: 169

Taylor J B 1981 Preconception clinics. British Medical Journal 283: 685

Tuck S M, Studd J W W, White J M, 1983 Pregnancy in sickle cell disease in the United Kingdom. British Journal of Obstetrics and Gynaecology 90: 112–7

Vessey M P, Wright N H, McPherson K, Wiggins P 1978 Fertility after stopping different methods of contraception. British Medical Journal 177: 265–67

Ward N I 1987 Placental element levels in relation to fetal development for obstetrically normal births: a study of 37 elements, evidence for effects of cadmium, lead, and zinc on fetal growth, and smoking as a source of cadmium. International Journal of Biosocial Research 9(1): 63–81

Williams R J 1973 Nutrition against disease. Bantam, New York

Witchells J 1984 Preconception care. Johnson & Johnson Baby Newsline No 33

Wood S M, Bexley L 1981 Prescribing in pregnancy. W B Saunders, London

Wynn M, Wynn A 1981 The importance of nutrition around the time of conception in the prevention of handicap. Applied Nutrition 1: 12–19

Zipper J A, Model M, Prager R 1969 Suppression of fertility by intrauterine copper and zinc in rabbits. American Journal of Obstetrics and Gynaecology 105: 529

■ Suggested further reading

Bamfield T 1989 Preparing for pregnancy. In Bennett V R, Brown L K (eds) Myles textbook for midwives (11th ed). Churchill Livingstone, Edinburgh

Chamberlain G, Lumley J 1986 Prepregnancy care – a manual for practice. John Wiley, Chichester

Daly H, Clarke P, Field J 1988 Diabetes care – a problem solving approach: 101–08. Heinemann, London

Harper P S 1984 Practical genetic counselling (2nd ed). John Wright, Bristol

Robarts J 1988 Preparing for pregnancy. Faber & Faber, London

Sweet R 1988 Mayes' midwifery – a textbook for midwives (11th ed): 55–61; 99–102; 115–25. Baillière Tindall, London

Chapter 2

The organisation of midwifery care

Rosemary Currell

When midwifery care entailed a more or less skilled woman in the village attending the confinements of her neighbours, little organisation was required. Now that midwifery care entails all women in the Western World being closely monitored throughout pregnancy, labour and the postnatal days by women who have highly developed clinical and interpersonal skills, organisation is a major concern for all involved. Georgopoulos (1972) describing the problems of hospital organisation states:

> However useful or necessary technological progress might be, it is not a substitute for social efficiency; technological innovation and improvements cannot compensate for obsolescence in the social-psychological sector and organisational arrangements on which the system relies.

The trend towards almost 100 per cent institutional deliveries in Britain and North America, together with the development of obstetric technology and Western parents' very high expectations of successful childbearing, have created very complex organisational problems within the maternity services. Shortcomings in maternity care have been examined by consumers, social scientists, doctors, and journalists as well as by midwives; sometimes in a rigorous and systematic way, and sometimes not. Many schemes to overcome these failings in the service have been suggested, tried and occasionally tested. Some of these will be examined here, and it will be suggested that the prevailing theme in the literature of 'continuity of care' as a cure for all the ills in the maternity services, is an imprecise and unhelpful concept. It will be argued that it could usefully be replaced by the concept of 'unity of care', and the application of this concept to clinical practice will be explored.

20

■ It is assumed that you are already aware of the following:

- The history of the midwifery services in the UK;
- The way in which maternity services are organised in your area;
- The midwifery process as applied to antenatal care and be familiar with the concepts of birthplans and individual programme planning;
- The different approaches in antenatal care which might be ideal for a woman in a low risk group pregnant for the second time, for a woman from the most prominent ethnic minority group in your area, and for a primigravida of 40 expecting twins.

■ The development of modern maternity care

Women have attended one another in childbirth since the beginning of history. Different cultures have always had different ways of supporting women and of institutionalising and ritualising childbirth. In the West it has been changes in the significance attached to childbirth, changes in the groups of people involved in the care of women, and changes in midwifery and obstetric practice which have led to an ever increasing complexity in the organisation of maternity care. The history of maternity care in Britain, and the development of the midwifery profession is well presented by Donnison (1977) in *Midwives and Medical Men*.

The major events which have contributed to the present organisation of maternity care include the following.

□ The founding of 'lying-in hospitals'

In the 18th and 19th centuries poorer women were admitted to the lying-in wards of the new hospitals in major cities. Infection was the first problem to become manifest as a result of delivering women in institutions instead of at home, and it has been followed by the long train of difficulties which has bedevilled the maternity services to this day (Donnison 1977).

□ The introduction of antenatal care

Antenatal care did not begin to develop until the early 20th century as medicine had very little to offer women before this time. The first British hospital antenatal clinic was opened in Edinburgh in 1915, and by 1935 it was estimated that 80 per cent of pregnant women in Britain were receiving some antenatal care. By this time also, the recommended intervals for antenatal examinations – at 16, 24, 28, 30, 32, 34 and 36 weeks of pregnancy, and then at weekly intervals to delivery – had become established. (See Oakley 1982, for a full account of the development of antenatal care.) This pattern of care is that which is still generally accepted and practised. It was challenged by Hall *et al* in 1980, and is still a matter for research and debate.

☐ The registration of midwives

The end of the 19th century saw the battle over the regulation of midwifery in Britain, which culminated in the first Midwives' Act in 1902. This act made midwifery the legitimate concern of both the midwifery and medical professions, but with the medical profession retaining some control over midwifery practice.

☐ Official policies and recommendations for the maternity services in Britain

Since the creation of the NHS in 1948, there have been a number of government reports and recommendations for maternity care (see pages 24–38). These have influenced the organisation of the service in a number of ways, and have therefore also influenced midwifery practice. The reports have reflected some of the prevailing philosophies of health care, and their effects on the maternity services will be discussed below.

■ The organisation of maternity care in Britain today

Four main patterns of maternity care have evolved in Britain today.

1. Home delivery – a woman receives all her care from a general practitioner and community midwives, possibly with a consultation with an obstetrician in the antenatal period.

2. Consultant unit care – a woman receives all her antenatal, labour and delivery, and early postnatal care from midwives and obstetric medical staff in a consultant unit.

3. Shared care – a woman receives an agreed part of her antenatal care from consultant unit staff and the rest from a GP and community midwife. She is delivered in the consultant unit, has her early postnatal care there and then returns to the care of her GP and community midwife.

4. GP unit care – a woman receives all her maternity care from a GP and either community midwives or community midwives and midwives attached to the GP unit.

Because not all GPs qualify for inclusion on the obstetric list, the doctor who gives a woman obstetric care may or may not be her own GP. She may transfer to the care of another GP just for her maternity care.

One major variation on these themes is the 'domino delivery scheme'. Here, a woman may have either shared care, or GP care in the antenatal period, and then be cared for during labour and delivery, and postnatally by a community midwife. This may take place in a consultant unit or a GP unit, and is usually combined with planned early transfer home.

Women may choose to have all their care from an independent midwife, or other private care from midwives and obstetricians at home or in an institution. Special organisational arrangements may be made for women with particular needs. These groups may include very young teenagers, women from ethnic minority groups, travellers, and women at special medical or obstetric risk. Schemes devised for some of these women will be discussed below.

■ A review of the literature

The literature of both the maternity services and midwifery care, is made up very largely of normative discourse by the author, or an historical review of a particular area or type of practice, or purely descriptive papers about a method of care which is either proposed or in use. We have to look further for hard evidence of the acceptability or effectiveness of any particular form of care, and for scientific testing of methods of care.

Research into the organisation of maternity and midwifery care has been carried out by midwives, obstetricians and GPs, epidemiologists, social scientists and politicians. A variety of research methods have been used. Governments have convened committees of inquiry who have taken evidence from experts, and recommended future policies. During the late 1970s and early 1980s consumer opinion of the maternity services was investigated. This was done principally by the Community Health Councils (CHCs), using quota samples of women receiving care in their area, and collecting data through the use of questionnaires (Garcia 1981). Detailed qualitative research has been carried out by social scientists into some of the issues raised by consumers, governments and professionals. The work of Graham (1980), and Macintyre (1982) on antenatal care are examples of this kind of research. There have been comparative studies, comparing one system of care with another (for example, Currell 1985); experimental studies which have looked at one area before and after the introduction of a change in care (for example Auld 1968; Metcalf 1981); and studies which have attempted to measure the success of a different method of care by introducing it alongside an existing system using those women as a control group (for example Thomas *et al* 1987). In some studies groups have been matched for significant factors. The randomised controlled trial is a favoured research method in medicine, and it has been used as a research method in midwifery care (for example Flint & Poulgeneris 1987). Research into the organisation of the maternity services has also used both retrospective and prospective methods (for example Klein *et al* 1983, 1985).

Midwifery research has sometimes focused on a particular aspect of care, such as breastfeeding, and then shown the effect that organisational factors have on clinical care (for example Houston 1981). Other researchers set out to study clinical problems in their organisational context (for example Ball 1981). Yet other researchers have focused on the organisation of care and revealed differences in clinical practice (for example Klein *et al* 1983). It is clear that clinical practice and organisational arrangements can never be completely disentangled.

☐ Government reports

Although government reports on the maternity services may not strictly be termed 'research', a review of the major reports will offer a partial explanation for the present organisation of the service. It will also reveal themes and preoccupations in the care of mothers and babies which run throughout the literature of the maternity services and continue to be subjects for discussion and research.

The National Health Service Act of 1946 created a tripartite system with care shared between hospitals, local authority health services and the general practitioner executive councils. The Guillebaud Committee (Ministry of Health 1955) found that the shared responsibility for the maternity services, made the service very complex, with duplication of effort and lack of co-ordination. The Guillebaud Committee therefore recommended a review of the organisation of the maternity services and this was undertaken by the Cranbrook Committee (Ministry of Health 1959). The Cranbrook Committee did not think it right, at that time, to place the service under the control of a single body, but its recommendations included the setting up of local maternity liaison committees and the use of maternity co-operation cards. The Committee recommended the provision of sufficient maternity beds for an average 70 per cent institutional confinement rate, and an assumed postnatal hospital stay of ten days. The situation changed very rapidly however, and was reviewed by the Peel Committee who reported in 1970.

Between 1955 and 1965 the number of hospital maternity beds rose by 15 per cent and the birth rate rose by 30 per cent. By 1968 hospital confinements had reached 80.8 per cent of the total births, and this was only being managed by a reduction in the length of postnatal stay. Forty-eight hour discharges from hospital had been introduced in some areas as a matter of expediency. It is important to note how changes in organisation can come about as the result of response to a practical difficulty rather than as the result of a changed philosophical concept or carefully planned research.

One of the issues in the organisation of maternity care raised by the Peel Committee (DHSS 1970) was that of continuity of care. The report stated:

> Continuity of care is a question raised several times in evidence and such a concept is indisputably a good one. We are concerned however that it should not be construed narrowly as a continuous personal relationship between the patient and only one midwife or doctor. Modern organisational trends such as the creation of health centres, the setting up of group practices and the introduction of off-duty rotas, are making this interpretation less and less appropriate.

It went on to recommend that care be provided by consultants, GPs and midwives, working in teams.

Increased hospital delivery rates obviously increased the significance of hospital routines for women, and 'The organisation of the in-patients' day' (DHSS 1976) contains some specific recommendations for maternity patients. These included creating a 'congenial and supportive atmosphere', a 'flexible attitude to care', and the formation of a common policy to 'help ensure continuity of care'.

The Short Report (HC 1980), is a major review of the maternity services in Britain. One hundred and fifty recommendations are made in the report, several of which have appeared in earlier documents. The report contains a chapter entitled 'Humanising the service', a theme which recurs constantly in the literature. The Committee also states: 'We recognise the difficulties of providing continuity of care throughout pregnancy and labour, but consider that a measure of it can be obtained by better organisation.' This again is an ill defined and unsupported promotion of continuity of care. The Maternity Services Advisory Committee was created as a result of the Short Report recommendations, and in its turn produced a three-part report, 'Maternity care in action (1982–4)'. This is a guide to good practice which again stresses the need for a flexible approach to care. It also refers to 'continuity of care' advocating a team approach. The Cumberlege Report – 'Neighbourhood nursing: a focus for care' (DHSS 1986) – included recommendations for the organisation and practice of community midwifery. Again, as the Guillebaud Committee had done in 1955, this committee identified the problems of poor communication and duplication of effort in the maternity services. It also identified the need for the service to be sensitive to the requirements of individuals and their families.

This brief review of some of the official reports of the maternity services in Britain has identified some common themes and problems. These may be summarised as follows:

● Changing work patterns brought about by the move to institutional deliveries and by changes in obstetric practice;

● The need to make optimum use of midwifery skills;

● The importance of good communications between all care givers, and between care givers and their clients;

● The need for a service which is flexible and sensitive to women's needs;

● Continuity of care;

● Adequate provision of facilities and resources;

● The desirability of all pregnant women receiving some care from a consultant obstetrician;

● The position of the GP in maternity care.

Debates and discussions about all these issues can be found in the professional journals and in the popular press, and some have been the subject of research.

□ CHC studies

Community health council (CHC) studies of the maternity services have been well reviewed by Garcia (1981), but it may be helpful to examine a few aspects of these studies here, as some of the issues they raise have been taken up for further research. The data collection methods used in these studies is usually self-administered questionnaires or sometimes interviews, but the response rate in some is very much lower than might be expected. It is usually thought that women are pleased to co-operate in work which might benefit other mothers and babies, but in the Bexley study (Bexley CHC 1979) the response rate was only 26.8 per cent and in West Surrey and North East Hampshire CHC (1979) study it was only 51 per cent. Most of these studies include women's views of their antenatal care, concentrate on the practical aspects of clinic visits and describe women's encounters with staff. Difficulties in communication are a common theme in these reports. The King's study (King's CHC 1978) suggested the creation of the post of 'Antenatal counsellor'. In the Islington study, Tunstall (1978) reports women's difficulties in obtaining information and says that women found seeing different doctors confusing. She states that, 'continuity of care is of major importance'. These reports were followed by more detailed research into some of these aspects of care.

□ Antenatal care

A major survey of women's views of antenatal care was carried out by O'Brien and Smith (1981). Two thousand, four hundred women were approached, with a response rate of 91 per cent. Women reported longer travelling times and longer waiting times at hospital visits than at visits to their GP, as women in the CHC studies had also done. They found that in both the hospital and GP visits, women who had received care from different people each time were less likely to say that their care was 'very good' than those who saw only one or two people throughout. They were also less likely to say that they felt able to discuss their worries or that what was happening was well explained. The authors suggest that continuity of care is an important factor in client satisfaction.

In answer to the question 'Why don't women attend for antenatal care?' Parsons and Perkins (1980) found in their study, firstly that the numbers of women who did not attend for antenatal care was much smaller than they had thought and, secondly, that they fell into three distinct groups: frightened teenagers, competent childbearers, and those with social problems. These are the same groups identified by O'Brien and Smith in their (1981) study as those who came late for antenatal care. It would appear from these findings that the vast majority of women have accepted the need to attend for antenatal care in spite of the dissatisfactions they may have with it. These studies suggest that improving antenatal clinics is not merely a matter of correcting administrative or comfort factors, as those who stay away may do so either because they are frightened of admitting to pregnancy or, judging by their previous experience of motherhood, may see no value in attending.

In a sociological study of pregnancy and motherhood, Graham (1980) suggests that the problems women face at this time are those of uncertainty about new or increased responsibilities. She found that women's positive attitudes to antenatal care were related to receiving reassurance about their own health and the health of their baby, and that their negative feelings were related to the strangeness of the patient role. Graham also describes the fragmented nature of clinic visits, and the lack of continuity, together with women's desire for more personal care, but she does not discuss continuity of care in any depth.

There have been studies which have looked at the content of care in antenatal clinics by using direct observational research methods. Macintyre (1982) interviewed in depth 50 women having a first baby. She found a lack of knowledge amongst them about the purpose of antenatal care, although the majority of them found it 'reassuring'. She also looked at the nature of the interviews between women and doctors in the clinics, and found that on average, the doctors spent 5.46 minutes with each woman, and that 37 per cent of women did not ask any questions at all. Macintyre suggests that it is more important to improve the quality of the care offered than it is to improve physical aspects of clinics, such as decor. Methven (1982) studied in detail the antenatal booking interview by midwives, and concluded that the organisation of care in clinics prevents women forming relationships with midwives. She shows how the midwifery process can be used to form a more satisfactory basis for this aspect of midwifery care (see also Chapter 3 in this volume, 'The antenatal booking interview' by Rosemary Methven).

In some areas, antenatal care has been specially designed for women with particular needs. For example Nunnerley (1985) describes a clinic for teenagers, and Butters (1987) describes an obstetric medical clinic for women with pregnancies at high risk. Davies (1988) describes the development of a neighbourhood centre on a council estate which both mothers and midwives use as a base. Antenatal care taken into the community has been the basis for a number of development projects (Heywood 1988).

□ Community clinics

Much of the 'action research' in maternity care has been in setting up community clinics. These take a variety of forms and have very similar aims. Some have assessed their results. The main aims of all these schemes are;

- To make antenatal care accessible to women;
- To reach groups with special needs;
- To make the clinics friendly and pleasant places to be;
- To make the best use of the skills of the practitioners;
- To improve perinatal outcomes for women and babies.

These programmes have been reviewed by Heywood (1988), who differentiates between those which are consultant hospital clinics taken to a peripheral location, and those which are community clinics attended by GPs and community midwives as well as consultant unit staff.

Perhaps the best known of these schemes is the Sighthill clinic, which was introduced in 1975 in Edinburgh, and involves GPs, community midwives, health visitors and a consultant obstetrician. The scheme of care is very structured, with assessment of women against a check list of risk factors and a pre-planned programme of management. Group discussions by the staff about client care are an important feature of the system. The perinatal mortality rate for the area has fallen since the introduction of the scheme, and the number of defaulters from the clinic is now very small. A similar system is described by Zander *et al* (1978), in which the consultant goes out to the GP's surgery. Here the authors make a positive statement that, 'there should be a continuing personal relationship between the patient and her professional adviser throughout pregnancy,' but this is not discussed in the context of a woman's total maternity care and midwives are not mentioned in this plan of antenatal care at all.

'An integrated community ante-natal clinic' is described by Thomas *et al* (1987). This clinic was held in a health centre and staffed by GPs, a community midwife and obstetric registrar. This care was compared with ordinary 'shared care'. The study group had more continuity from the hospital doctor than the control group, and found him easier to talk to. This finding relates to one individual obstetric registrar, however, and may be a consequence of his personality, rather than a consequence of altered structures in the clinic organisation. The authors report administrative difficulties with this clinic. The burden appears to have fallen on the community midwife who was the least satisfied member of staff in the clinic.

The community clinic at Easterhouse has also been carefully evaluated (Reid *et al* 1983). The project began with a pilot study to identify the aspects of antenatal care which women wanted changed. The problems of travelling, waiting, the quality of doctor/client communications, and a desire for more continuity of care were identified. The clinic was set up on a housing estate, with both hospital and community staff, and was compared with the hospital clinic. Although they found that the women in the peripheral clinic saw a significantly lower number of doctors during their antenatal care, they did not find a significant difference in the quality of doctor/client communications. The fact that 85 per cent of the women in one group and 74 per cent in the other reported that, on the day of the research interview, they did not have any discussion with a member of the clinic staff other than the doctor, is very important for midwives. It may have been that they truly did have no discussion at all with other staff, or that the quality of the encounters was such that it had no significance for them. This study attempts to identify ways in which the organisation of maternity care can be improved for the consumer. The authors conclude:

> The results of the project show that the mere removal of a clinic to a different location will achieve little in terms of improved communications if many of the structural and attitudinal features of the clinic remain unchanged.

The study shows the need for the encounters between women, midwives and doctors, in all aspects of maternity care, to be examined more closely. All these studies show that the factors which women are able to articulate as problems, and to which midwives and doctors have responded, may not be the real failings of antenatal care.

☐ The organisation of midwifery care

A number of schemes have been developed or adapted by midwives in an attempt to provide total patient care. In 1968, Auld described a system of hospital-based team nursing (involving nurses, students and auxiliaries as well as midwives) which was introduced into a maternity unit to replace a system of task allocation. Although most of the staff were pleased with the team nursing, Auld could find no differences in the mothers' reports of the two systems. In another study (Auld 1976), the same author carried out activity sampling of midwives' work in order to establish a basis for staffing levels. Auld again asserts the advantages of organising midwifery work on a team basis, but the study is not able to demonstrate positively the benefits she suggests. Her observations do show the complex and fragmented nature of midwifery work in hospital. Auld also makes a most important observation about midwifery practice which may be one of the reasons why organisational changes in antenatal care have been relatively unsuccessful. She states:

> The ability to provide psychological support is so much part of the individual's own make-up, that for some it is automatic, but for others, even the provision of more time to allow them to carry out their nursing function to its utmost would still fail to elicit the psychological support which is so important to most patients.

Metcalf (1981), reported the results of another study designed to determine whether a system of patient allocation, instead of task allocation, would improve mothers' and midwives' satisfaction with care. During this study, observations were made and mothers and staff satisfaction were measured before, during and after the change was made. The author states that continuity of care was the aim of the change. Metcalf reports little change in the observed work carried out by the staff, although she stresses that her observations were quantitative rather than qualitative. She found little evidence that patient allocation improved job satisfaction for staff. She found mothers satisfied with both systems, although they did perceive more nurse-patient continuity after the change. There was no significant difference in the number of mothers who felt they had been treated as 'individuals' before or after the change. Metcalf concludes that it is not essential to have a system of patient allocation in order to give 'individualised' care.

The 'Know your midwife scheme' (Flint & Poulgeneris 1987) is a study designed to test the feasibility of a small team of midwives giving total care to a group of women, and to test the advantages of continuity of care. This was a randomised controlled trial comparing conventional hospital care for low risk women with care given to an experimental group of low risk women. In the experimental group, women received care during pregnancy, labour and the puerperium from a team of four midwives. This pattern of care is similar to that in the Oxford GP unit (Klein et al 1983) and the

Lexden GP unit group (Currell 1985) which are discussed in more detail below.

In the 'Know your midwife' (KYM) study, the randomisation of the women to the two groups appears to have worked well. Women were given self-administered questionnaires at 37 weeks gestation, two days postnatally and six weeks postnatally. On some measures of satisfaction there were significant differences between the two groups. For example, a statistically significant number of the KYM group felt that their midwives showed a personal interest in them, but there was no statistical difference in the numbers in the two groups who found midwives 'friendly', or in those who felt questions were answered well, or in the numbers who thought midwives encouraged more questions than doctors. It is likely that an observer effect was operating here, as when women were invited to take part in the KYM scheme, they were sent a letter which read, '. . . we shall be seeing only a small number of women and we hope you will get to know us as friends and that we shall get to know you well'. Here is the stated intention by the midwives to know this group of women well, so it is hardly surprising that the women in this group felt that the midwives took a personal interest in them.

There were no statistically significant differences between the two groups in the numbers of women who intended to breastfeed, in the help women said they received from staff postnatally, or in their confidence with their babies. At two days postnatally, more of the women in the control group than in the KYM group thought that labour had been a 'wonderful' or 'enjoyable' experience, although this does not reach statistical significance. At six weeks, however, significantly more of the KYM group thought labour had been a wonderful experience. It is interesting to note this shift, and it may be that women's immediate reaction to labour is the one which is less open to influence – by family, friends or professionals. The authors report differences between the two groups in factors such as electronic fetal monitoring, use of analgesia, positions for delivery, the amount of time spent walking in labour, and babies put to the breast immediately. All these factors may be related to the practice of individual midwives, rather than to organisational aspects of care or to women's positive choices for labour. However, the KYM scheme does show that it is possible to organise care for a group of women in this way and that it can achieve good clinical results.

A retrospective study was carried out by Klein *et al* (1983) comparing care for low risk women in a shared care system and in an integrated GP unit system. The midwifery staff were organised in the GP unit in a similar way to those in the KYM scheme. The authors showed that short term clinical outcomes were as good for the women in the GP unit as for those in the shared care system, and in some instances better. This study shows how organisation, local policies and local geographical factors can all affect the care women receive. In the study area, the GP unit can only be used by doctors whose practices fall within a limited radius of the consultant unit.

This means that women at low risk living outside this catchment area do not have access to this system of care. The different organisational arrangements for the two groups also meant that the women in the GP unit group could be visited at home by their community midwives in early labour, and thus spent less time in hospital in unestablished labour than the women in the shared care group. As in the KYM scheme, the authors report more intervention and greater use of analgesia for the women in the shared care system, and suggest that this may be in part the result of difficulties for hospital midwives in caring for women at both high and low risk, and the more complex relationships which hospital midwives have with other professionals.

This study was followed by a prospective study (Klein *et al* 1985), in which women in the two systems of care were also asked about their attitudes to the maternity care they received, and about breastfeeding in the first three months. They found women in both groups to be generally pleased with the care they had received. There were some differences in their views, with the general trend in favour of the GP unit, but these did not reach statistical significance and had largely disappeared by three months postpartum. Dissatisfactions with either system were rare.

The organisation of health care in the USA is very different from that in Britain, and comparative studies of different organisational pratices within the USA have been carried out. For example, Wilner *et al* (1981) compared the care and the clinical outcomes for mothers and babies receiving care in private 'fee for service' practices with those receiving care in a health maintenance organisation based on payment through insurance. They found outcomes and quality of care to be similar in both systems, though the caesarean section rate was lower in the health maintenance organisation group. Organising care by financial criteria does not therefore necessarily produce different outcomes for mothers and babies.

Another comparative study of shared care and GP unit care, and also home delivery care, was undertaken by this author (Currell 1985). The study was carried out in two areas of the south of England in order to test the hypothesis that the organisational patterns of maternity care would be found along a continuum with continuity of care at one end and fragmented care at the other. It was also hypothesised that the women who received the greatest degree of continuity of care would be the most satisfied, and that those who received the most fragmented care would be the least satisfied. It was also expected that the midwives giving the greatest degree of continuity of care would have the greatest job satisfaction, and those giving the most fragmented care the least. Considerable fragmentation of care was found in all the groups except for the care of a very few of the women who had a home delivery. No statistically significant differences were found between the groups in such factors as, for example, the support women felt they had received during labour, whether or not they thought procedures or what to expect during pregnancy had been well explained to them, the help they experienced from professionals in the postnatal period, feeling 'weepy' postnatally, and their sources of information about babycare. Both praise and criticisms of midwives and their care were found in all the patterns of care.

Although the two consultant units in the study differed considerably in size – one with approximately 5500 deliveries each year, and the other with approximately 2000 deliveries a year at the time of the study – the number of staff women met in the postnatal wards in the two units were very similar. In one of the two areas, the GP unit was an integrated unit in the consultant unit, and the number of staff women met in the postnatal wards there was the same for both groups. This study shows that maternity care is very complex for the great majority of women in Britain whatever organisational pattern of care is used. It shows that 'continuity of care' is an elusive concept and, as other studies have shown, that satisfaction with maternity care is dependent on factors other than how midwives and doctors organise their work. The study also failed to show greater job satisfaction for midwives in one organisational pattern of care rather than another. However, the study did show that both mothers and midwives felt satisfaction with care which resulted in the resolution of a problem of some kind, a breastfeeding problem for example. It is suggested, therefore, that it is effective problem solving which produces satisfaction, and that this is most likely to be achieved not by reorganising the areas in which midwives work, but by focusing on every encounter between mothers and midwives, wherever it takes place, and whether the mother and midwife have met before or not.

The midwifery process is a tool which has been used in attempts to improve midwifery care, and has usually been implemented with a system of either patient allocation or team midwifery. Descriptive accounts of the use of the midwifery process are given by, for example, Adams *et al* (1981), Bryar and Strong (1983) and Tiran and Nunnerley (1986). The authors all report a more flexible approach to care and better understanding of women's needs, from this approach to care, and describe its usefulness as a teaching aid for students. They found difficulties in implementing these systems because of the problems of staff rotas, staff mix, the increased time needed with the mothers and the increased paperwork.

Midwives have examined specific problems in maternity care and found organisational implications in their solutions. Houston and Howie (1981) showed how extra, systematic home support for breastfeeding mothers appeared to help women continue feeding for longer and to postpone the introduction of supplementary feeding. This study shows that recognising a problem women may have, and offering practical help and support in an organised way to overcome it, is a most effective form of maternity care.

Ball (1981) examined the effects of patterns of maternity care on the emotional needs of mothers. She found that women's levels of emotional satisfaction or distress, measured by the 'family bond score' constructed during the research, were significantly related to social class, perceptions of postnatal care and memories of the birth itself. The women in social class IV were identified as the most vulnerable, which is a reminder both of the importance for women of factors operating outside the maternity services, and the difficulties which some women may have in making the service work to their best advantage. Ball identified conflicting advice in the postnatal period as a major difficulty for women. Again, individual and carefully planned care, which elicits each woman's problems and responds effectively, must reduce the difficulties women perceive from apparently conflicting advice from professionals. Ball stressed the importance of the emotional support which midwives are able to give to women, and the great need for good communications in maternity care.

■ Recommendations on the basis of currently available evidence

As maternity care in the West has gradually been brought into hospitals and institutions, so it has become increasingly complex and increasingly technical. Confusion about the aims of the service, and about the reasonable expectations which consumers might have of the service, have led to frustration and unhappiness for both recipients and providers of care. There has been a desire to 'humanise' the service and to restore the place of the individual and at the same time, to improve the clinical outcomes for mothers and babies. The research studies discussed above have all, in some way, sought to identify the factors which make the service ineffective and unacceptable to mothers. Some have changed the organisation of care in attempts to improve it, but all with limited success. For example, Hall *et al* (1980) showed the deficiencies of clinical antenatal care. Reid *et al* (1983) have shown that merely changing a clinic location and reducing the number of staff with whom individual women have contact will not by itself improve women's satisfaction with their care. Metcalf (1981) has shown that changing midwives' work patterns from task allocation to team midwifery will not alone change women's perceptions of the care they have received.

☐ Continuity of care

Continuity of care is a concept which has been constantly cited as a means for improving maternity care. Nowhere in the literature, however, has it been adequately defined or analysed in depth. Some research, for example Flint *et al* (1987) and Currell (1985), has tried to demonstrate the expected benefits of continuity of care, but with very limited success. It is possible that the ideals of 'continuity of care' have never been met, even when women received all their maternity care from a community midwife. Gregory (1923), in *The midwife: her book*, describes a postnatal visit at the time of World War I, which ends with the mother saying: 'I did like that young nurse as used to come to you and me. She was kind and gentle when baby was coming, though always in such a bustle when she came afterwards. There, I daresay they gave her too much to do.'

Care that is ineffective, inappropriate, unacceptable, or simply wrong, can be of no value even if it is given under the umbrella of 'continuity'. Organisation in the maternity services therefore needs to look both deeper and beyond the idea of 'continuity of care' if real progress is to be made.

□ Focused care

It is evident from the literature that effective problem solving with mothers makes for satisfaction with care. Houston and Howie (1981) show this for breastfeeding mothers. Parboosingh and Kerr (1982) report the benefits for women and the very low default rate in the Sighthill project, where women attend for antenatal care in a clinic close to their home reducing the problems of long, difficult and expensive journeys to hospital. Women report satisfaction with antenatal care where they feel that they have been given reassurance and their questions have been answered (Currell 1985). Perhaps, therefore, it is the individual encounters between mothers and midwives which need to be examined closely. Kratz (1978) in her research into the care given by community nurses to the longterm sick, offers a means of studying these encounters. She describes four kinds of care: focused care, semi-focused care, semi-diffuse care and diffuse care. The first and the last of these will be considered here. Kratz describes focused care as being care in which: 'the aim of care is known and the care valued. The care given corresponds to the observed needs of patients.' She describes diffuse care as being care in which: 'the aim of care is not known and the care is not valued'.

The literature shows that where there is a specific problem (such as a breastfeeding problem) which is identified and solved there is mutual satisfaction for mother and midwife. This care has been understood and valued by both of them and could therefore be defined as 'focused care'. Currell (1985) shows how women are usually delighted with the midwifery care they receive in labour and at delivery, whether they knew the midwife beforehand or not. This finding suggests that this care is well understood and valued by both mothers and midwives and, again, could be defined as 'focused care'. In the antenatal period it has been seen that where women's need for reassurance has been identified and met, they report satisfaction. In the brief and disjointed antenatal visits which have also been described in the literature, however, it appears that in the absence of any well defined problems, much of antenatal care may be defined as 'diffuse care'. Research (for example Graham 1980) suggests that much of antenatal care and its aims are not well understood, and the care is not valued.

It is recommended, therefore, that all maternity care should be examined to ensure that it is focused care, and therefore effective and satisfying to both mothers and midwives. It must be realised that focused care is more than 'problem solving' in midwifery care. Focused care may mean helping a mother whose baby has difficulty in 'fixing' at the breast – a well defined and recognised problem which can be seen to have been resolved when breastfeeding is established. Focused care, however, may also mean listening to a woman recount the delivery of her stillborn baby. This is not a 'problem' which can be 'solved', but it is a need for sensitive care from the midwife, and care which can be emotionally helpful for the mother, even though it may have no obvious outcome.

☐ Care and cure

Where mothers and midwives see the need for physical intervention to solve a problem, or an obvious need for support, as in labour, care appears to be successful and the rewards immediate for everyone. Any attempt to focus midwifery care, and to consider carefully all encounters between women and midwives will, however, soon reveal women's needs for supportive care which is less obvious and provides less instant gratification for the midwife. The dilemma of 'care and cure' is well documented in all aspects of health care. Klein *et al* (1983) identified the difficulties for consultant unit midwives giving both technical and supportive care to women at both high and low risk in labour. Wilson (1971) states that, 'care is a concept that does not have to be validated by clinical results'. Perhaps now more than ever before, midwives must be able to hold the balance between giving good, safe clinical care, and giving the emotional and psychological support that women need. Talking and listening to women should be seen as valued care in any maternity care organisation, but Metcalf (1981) reported that midwives did not approach women on the postnatal wards without having a specific task.

☐ Unity of care

Personal continuity of midwifery care is undoubtedly pleasant and rewarding, as this author will testify. When continuity of care is discussed in relation to the maternity services, however, it is primarily describing characteristics of the working life of the care providers. It is care directed towards mothers and babies, but it is the professional care which is being described, not the total experience of the woman and her family. Writers may say that it is care which women 'like' or 'want', but descriptions of 'continuity of care' are descriptions of the way professionals organise their work, not a description or definition of the nature or quality of any care that may be given within that particular organisational framework.

The Oxford English Dictionary definition of 'continuity' is simply, 'the state of being continuous', but the definition of 'unity' is, 'oneness, being one or single, or individual, being formed of parts that constitute a whole, due interconnection and coherence of parts . . . thing that forms a complex whole . . . harmony, concord between persons'. To talk of 'unity of care', then, must be to turn away from the caregivers and towards the woman herself. If we aim to provide a service which gives unity of care to each woman and her family, she becomes the centre of the service and of the organisation. Care must be organised in an individual and focused way, so that all encounters with staff contribute to the whole. This approach to the organisation of care will inevitably take into account the woman and her expectations beyond the limits of the maternity services. It will place the midwife in her true role of being 'with woman', as a facilitator, helping the woman to achieve her own goals for herself and her baby.

□ **Dependency**

In any attempt to organise a system of maternity care in which personal continuity between midwives and mothers is attempted, it should be remembered that several authors (for example Reid *et al* 1983; Currell 1985; Thomas *et al*, 1987) report women feeling 'let down' and 'deserted' if their expectations about one particular person being available or present are not fulfilled. The nature of these relationships needs further research before such systems are introduced. Disappointment is one thing, but it is no part of the midwife's role to create dependency. The cost of excessive personal demands on staff should also be evaluated. It would be important to know exactly what contribution was made to any of the research findings discussed above by the personality of some of the individual professionals who are attempting to provide continuity of care. Again, more research is needed into the nature of the emotional support women may need from the maternity services.

The literature has shown much innovative work carried out to meet local needs and the needs of special groups. It is clear that there is no right organisational pattern of maternity care. It must be organised to meet local, geographical and demographic needs, and must give the highest possible level of clinical care to all women. The implications from some of the research are that much of the care for women at low obstetric risk should be given by midwives. Care must be organised to meet each woman's personal wishes and convenience as far as possible. The organisation must be able to meet the training needs of midwives and doctors, and all these criteria could be met in many different ways.

A philosophy which may be helpful when considering the organisation of a midwifery service is that discussed by Campbell (1984) in *Moderated love: a theology of professional care*. In this work, Campbell describes how professional care is one response to the complexities and fragmentation which characterise our society. He describes the ambiguities implicit in professional caring, which the research literature has also shown. Indeed, the striving for 'continuity of care' may well be seen as an expression of this confusion. Campbell considers the work of doctors, nurses and social workers, but his description of how 'moderated love' may be expressed in nursing may be more readily understood by midwives. He considers tension between cure and care, between 'being with and doing to', and suggests nursing as 'skilled companionship'. He uses the imagery of a journey:

> Companionship arises from a chance meeting and it is terminated when the joint purpose which keeps companions together no longer obtains. The good companion is someone who shares freely, but does not impose, allowing others to make their own journey.

He goes on to discuss moderated love saying there is a detachment about it which is a protection for the client. He stresses that there is not equality in the relationship between client and care provider, but that there is mutuality. It may be that the idea of mutuality is helpful in the provision of a service which meets the needs of women first, and also provides satisfaction for those who work within the organisation.

■ Practice check

The following six tests might be applied to any system of maternity care.

- *Availability* – does the system provide a service for all who need it?

- *Accessibility* – is it possible for all who need the service to make use of it easily?

- *Acceptability* – is the service provided in a way which is congenial to those who need it?

- *Effectiveness* – does the service meet its own stated aims and identified needs of those it seeks to serve?

- *Efficiency* – does the service make the best use of all available resources, including the resources of its consumers?

- *Economy* – are there sufficient resources available to provide a service which meets all the criteria above?

■ References

Adams M, Armstrong-Esther C, Bryar R, Duberley J, Strong G, Ward E 1981 Trial run. Nursing Mirror 153(15): 32–5

Auld M 1968 Team nursing in a maternity hospital. Midwife and Health Visitor 4 (6): 242–45; 4 (6): 302–05

Auld M 1976 How many nurses? RCN, London

Ball J 1981 Effect of present patterns of maternity care on the emotional needs of mothers. Midwives Chronicle Part 1 – 94 (1120): 150–4; Part 2 – 94 (1121): 198–202; Part 3 – 94 (1122): 231–33

Bexley C H C 1979 Report of a survey of maternity services in Bexley Health District. London

Boddy K, Parboosingh J, Shepherd C 1978 A schematic approach to pre-natal care. Department of Obstetrics and Gynaecology, Edinburgh University

Bryar R, Strong G 1983 Trial run – continued. Nursing Mirror 155 (41): 45–48

Butters L 1987 The midwife and high-risk pregnancies. Midwives Chronicle 100 (1194): 199– 202

Campbell A V 1984 Moderated love: a theology of professional care. SPCK, London

Currell R A 1985 Continuity and fragmentation in maternity care. Unpublished M.Phil dissertation, University of Exeter

Davies J 1988 Cowgate Neighbourhood Centre – a preventative health care venture shared by midwives and social workers. Midwives Chronicle 101 (1200): 4–7

DHSS 1970 Domiciliary midwifery and maternity bed needs (Peel Report). HMSO, London

DHSS 1976 The organisation of the in-patient's day. HMSO, London

DHSS 1986 Neighbourhood nursing: a focus for care (Cumberlege Report). HMSO, London

Donnison J 1977 Midwives and medical men: a history of inter-professional rivalries and women's rights. Heinemann, London

Flint C Poulgeneris P 1987 The 'Know your midwife' report. Privately printed; available from 49 Peckarmans Wood, Sydenham Hill, London SE26 6RZ

Garcia J 1981 Findings on ante-natal care from community health council studies. National Perinatal Epidemiology Unit, Oxford

Georgopoulos B 1972 The problem of hospital organisation. In Organisation Research on Health Institutions. Institute of Social Research, UGA

Graham H 1980 Having a baby. Unpublished PhD thesis, University of York

Gregory A 1923 The midwife: her book. Hodder and Stoughton, London

Hall M Chng P, MacGillivray I 1980 Is routine ante-natal care worthwhile? Lancet ii(8185): 78–80

Heywood A 1988 Review of other community antenatal schemes in Great Britain. Community antenatal programme evaluation reports No 4. City and Hackney Health Authority, London

House of Commons Social Services Committee (HC) 1980 Report on perinatal and neonatal mortality (Short Report). HMSO, London

Houston M J, Howie P W 1981 Home support for the breast-feeding mother. Midwife, Health Visitor and Community Nurse 17(9):378–82

Kings C H C 1978 Report on maternity care in the King's Health District. London

Klein M, Lloyd I, Redman C, Bull M, Turnbull A 1983 A comparison of low-risk women booked for delivery in two different systems of care – shared care and GPU. British Journal of Obstetrics and Gynaecology 90(2): 118–28

Klein M, Elbourne D, Lloyd I 1985 A prospective study comparing the experience of low risk women booked for delivery in two systems of maternity care. Royal College of General Practitioners, London

Kratz C 1978 Care of the long term sick in the community. Churchill Livingstone, Edinburgh

Macintyre S 1982 Communications between pregnant women and their medical and midwifery attendants. Midwives Chronicle 95(1138): 387–94

Maternity Services Advisory Committee 1984–1985 Maternity care in action, Parts I, II and III. HMSO, London

Metcalf C 1981 Patient allocation in a maternity ward. Paper given at the Research and the Midwife conference, London 1981

Methven R 1982 The ante-natal booking interview: recording an obstetric history or relating with a mother-to-be? Paper given at the Research and the Midwife conference, London 1982

Ministry of health 1955 Report of the Committee of Enquiry into the cost of the National Health Service (Guillebaud Report). HMSO, London

Ministry of Health 1959 Report of the Maternity Services Committee (Cranbrook Report). HMSO, London

Nunnerley R 1985 Teenage dilemma. Midwives Chronicle 98(1172): 244–48

Oakley A 1982 The origins of antenatal care. In Enkin M, Chalmers I (eds) Effectiveness and satisfaction in antenatal care. Spastics International Medical Publications, London

O'Brien M, Smith C 1981 Women's views and experience of antenatal care. Practitioner 225: 123–26

Parboosingh J, Kerr M 1982 Innovation in the role of obstetric hospitals in prenatal care. In Enkin M, Chalmers I (eds) Effectiveness and satisfaction in antenatal care. Spastics International Publications, London

Parsons W, Perkins E 1980 Why don't women attend for ante-natal care? Leverhulme Health Educational Production, Occasional Paper No 23. University of Nottingham

Reid M, Gutteridge S, McIlwaine G M 1983 A comparison of the delivery of ante-natal care between a hospital and a peripheral clinic. Social Paediatric and Obstetric Research Unit, University of Glasgow/SHHD, Edinburgh

Thomas H, Draper J, Field S, Hare M 1987 Evaluation of an integrated community antenatal clinic. Journal of the Royal College of General Practitioners 37: 544–47

Tunstall S 1978 Experiencing childbirth: a survey of 40 Islington women. Islington CHC, London

West Surrey/North East Hampshire CHC 1979 Survey of maternity services in the West Surrey/North East Hampshire District. West Surrey/North East Hampshire CHC, Farnborough

Wilner S, Schoenbaum S C, Monson R R, Winickoff R N 1981 A comparison of the quality of maternity care between a health-maintenance organisation and fee for service practices. New England Journal of Medicine 304(13): 784–87

Wilson M 1971 The hospital – a place of truth: a study of the role of the hospital chaplain. University of Birmingham Institute for the Study of Worship and Religious Architecture, Birmingham

Zander L, Lee-Jones M, Fisher C 1978 The role of the primary health care team in the management of pregnancy. In Kitzinger S, Davis J (eds) The place of birth. Oxford Medical Publications, Oxford

■ Suggested further reading

Donnison J 1977 Midwives and medical men. Heinemann, London

Dowling S 1983 Health for a change: the provision of preventive health care in pregnancy and early childhood. Child Poverty Action Group in association with the National Extension College, London

Enkin M, Chalmers I (eds) 1982 Effectiveness and satisfaction in ante-natal care. Spastics International Medical Publictions, London

Enkin M, Keirse M J N C, Chalmers I (eds) 1989 A guide to effective care in pregnancy and childbirth. Oxford University Press, Oxford

Kitzinger S, Davis J A (eds) 1978 The place of birth. Oxford University Press, Oxford

Phaff J M L 1986 Perinatal health services in Europe: searching for better childbirth. Croom Helm, London

Chapter 3

The antenatal booking interview

Rosemary C. Methven

The traditional practice of entering details of a mother's 'booking history' on her obstetric record during the first visit to antenatal clinic is giving way to a much broader understanding of the scope and purpose of this first encounter between mother and midwife. Different strategies are being employed so that the antenatal booking interview can become a two-way giving and receiving of information in order that the mother and her partner can plan care with the midwife which is appropriate to their individual needs and expectations during pregnancy, labour and the postnatal period. The computerisation of obstetric records, experimental schemes where mothers carry their own maternity notes and changes in the organisation of antenatal care in general, have all affected the conduct and content of the antenatal booking interview.

This interaction between mother and midwife is considered to be the key element in developing a relationship between them and for determining the quality and effectiveness of a mother's subsequent maternity care.

■ It is assumed that you are already aware of the following:

- What information is essential, and what desirable, to obtain from a mother and her partner in order to plan their care during pregnancy and childbirth;

- The five main categories of question types and the way in which these should be used during a clinical interview (de Julia 1980);

- The techniques involved in conducting a clinical interview (Maguire & Rutter 1976; Open University 1979);

42

- Which skills are needed to develop a rapport with a mother and the significance of non-verbal communication (Smith & Bass 1982);

- How to design a care plan using the nursing/midwifery process or planned individualised care based on a suitable framework or model of care;

- Any protocols or policies operating within your own health district which may be relevant to the care and management of a mother and her partner during pregnancy, labour or the postnatal period.

■ The booking interview: a critical appraisal of relevant research literature

Ballantyne (1862–1923) has been credited with initiating antenatal care in Britain (Oakley 1983), but even in the 1930s many mothers still felt it was necessary to book a midwife only for the delivery itself (Towler and Bramall 1986). However, pressure from obstetricians, coupled with a shortage of facilities, eventually encouraged mothers to come to antenatal clinics during pregnancy so that they could be sure of booking a hospital bed for the birth of their baby. Consequently the first antenatal visit has come to be known as the booking clinic. During this visit the condition of the mother is assessed and the most appropriate place for the birth of her baby ascertained.

The 1978 edition of *Notices Concerning a Midwife's Code of Practice* stated: 'when in professional attendance on a maternity case, a midwife must as soon as practicable, interview the patient and take her history' (CMB 1978). Thus, the midwife's traditional role of recording obstetric information about a mother at the time of booking received official sanction irrespective of the place where her baby would eventually be born.

☐ The booking interview defined

A definition of the antenatal booking interview however is not clear cut, even though Fawdry and Mutch (1986) contend that 'recording an antenatal booking history is a relatively standard procedure'. Midwives see this interaction between mother and midwife as the first step in initiating that special relationship which characterises the uniqueness of midwifery practice (Walker 1976; Methven 1982a, 1989).

The establishment of risk factors is the purpose of the booking interview identified by both Savage (1980) and Symonds (1980). Chng *et al* (1980) consider that the antenatal booking interview is an opportunity to:

> review the medical and obstetric history of the pregnant woman, make a physical examination, perform appropriate investigations,

arrange suitable antenatal care for the rest of pregnancy, and book confinement in a setting with the facilities and professional expertise likely to be necessary. Advice on diet, alcohol consumption, and other health matters may be given and any problems discussed.

Thomson (1980), however, says of the midwifery history:

I do not mean the current form filling exercise, I mean the woman's physical, social, psychological and emotional state are assessed and on this assessment her needs are defined, care is then planned on the basis of this assessment.

Thus, in its narrowest sense, the antenatal booking interview may be regarded as merely obtaining and recording that information required by the obstetric case notes (Methven 1982a, 1989). By contrast, in its broadest sense, the interview is conceived as an opportunity for the midwife to discuss parents' expectations for childbirth and its management in pregnancy, labour and the postnatal period, and plan care accordingly.

☐ Content of the antenatal booking interview

The type and amount of information which may be given to parents and the range of decisions which may be made by a midwife will depend on the individual policies operating within any health authority as well as the location of the interview itself. Increasingly, this interview is being undertaken by midwives in the mother's own home preparatory to a conventional booking visit at the maternity hospital. Some would see the midwife as the initial point of contact for any mother who is expecting a baby, especially if her baby is to be born at home (ARM 1986; RCM 1987).

The traditional concept of a booking history is usually confined to recording information about those topics which are printed on the antenatal case notes. Midwives use these as a guide when questioning a mother about her medical, surgical, obstetric, social and family history as well as her present pregnancy. Methven (1982a, 1989) found that mothers were always questioned about these identified topics but subject areas which did not appear on the case notes were usually not discussed. She demonstrated that, in consequence, the format of the mother's antenatal case notes dictated not only the content of the booking history but also the order of questions and the way in which they were asked. Topics which were not printed on the case notes were usually not discussed with the mother, and if they did arise during the course of conversation, they were not recorded because there was nowhere appropriate to write them down.

As most case notes are designed by medical staff, the traditional booking history was found to consist of little more than obtaining an obstetric record. The element of initiating a relationship with a mother-to-be was lacking entirely (Methven 1982a).

☐ **Research related to the booking history**

Having analysed the content of 40 booking histories, Methven (1989) concluded that further research was needed to determine just what information was required in order that a mother's midwifery care could be satisfactorily planned.

Fawdry and Mutch (1986) undertook a similar exercise on the antenatal case notes of 41 teaching hospitals in the UK. Five hundred and seventy-one items were identified from these cases notes, which highlighted 'a tendency to collect data without sufficient evidence of their value'. Fawdry and Mutch go on to comment:

> although some reference to smoking occurred in 28 records (71%) there was little emphasis on alcohol consumption (15%), diet (2.5%) or domestic support (12%). Apart from the mother's intention regarding infant feeding (51%), few case notes prompted questions on personal attitudes or wishes of the expectant mother. Only four hospitals provided space for the mother's comments on epidural analgesia. None asked about her preferences in respect of alternative birth positions.

Methven's study also demonstrated that the midwifery relevance of obstetric items was not ascertained which meant that the quality of the mothers' subsequent care was likely to be deficient.

☐ **The booking interview as an assessment for planning care**

Methven's study compared the content and quality of a traditional booking history with a nursing process style of assessment based on a model of care (Orem 1980) undertaken on the same woman, (Methven 1986a, 1989). Although there are identifiable weaknesses in the research design of this part of the study, it nevertheless indicates quite clearly that use of an appropriate nursing/midwifery framework for the booking interview significantly increases both the quality of the interaction between mother and midwife and the relevance of the information obtained as a foundation on which the mother's maternity care can be subsequently planned. Bryar (1988) endorses this.

Specific models for midwifery are currently being developed (Mayes 1987; Midgley 1988; Hughes & Goldstone 1989; Crichton 1989); and this represents a significant step forward in the development of midwifery as a professional discipline (Green 1985) as well as going some way to meeting those needs identified by consumers themselves. It should be appreciated, however, that a care plan (Wilson 1988) or care card (Hope 1983) based on a framework of nursing or midwifery care, is not the same as a birthplan (Crook 1988). The midwifery process, or planned individualised care using a care plan, has been well documented by Whitfield (1983) and Heath *et al* (1986).

☐ Conduct of the booking interview

In the UK, interviewing is usually associated with selection for a job, although elsewhere the concept of a clinical interview is well established (de Julia 1980). It is described by Marriner (1979) as 'a method of learning about people through purposeful, goal-directed conversation'. McFarlane and Castledine (1982) consider it to be one of the 'most skilled nursing functions'.

Sadly, Macintyre's observation in an antenatal clinic concluded that the booking interview was perceived 'simply as a routine to be got through, the content being more important than the form' (Macintyre 1978). Methven's (1982b) analysis of 40 booking interviews undertaken in four different maternity hospitals showed that the mean duration of this interaction between mother and midwife was 20 minutes although a range of 5–35 minutes was recorded.

The history taking exercise formed a small proportion of the total time spent by mothers at booking clinic, which usually lasted between two and a half and three and a quarter hours. The average contact between mother and obstetrician at booking clinic was less than eight minutes, ranging between a minimum of just two minutes and a maximum of 25 minutes. However, as these latter figures are based on only eight visits, they cannot be considered representative, even though they were undertaken in four different maternity hospitals (Methven 1982b).

It is considered that a fresh approach to teaching the skills necessary for obtaining information from a mother in a reliable and consistent manner may also help to raise the booking interview from its currently perceived position as a low status task (Methven 1982a).

☐ Interview technique

The model developed by Maguire and Rutter (1976) to teach medical students how to interview patients in order to obtain a medical history has relevance for the conduct of the antenatal booking interview. Similarly, interview skills listed by the Open University (1979) form a helpful structure for midwives wishing to undertake such an interview with mothers.

These criteria were used as the framework for analysis in Methven's study. She found it hard to observe any attempt by midwives to develop a rapport with mothers or evidence of putting them at ease before beginning the information gathering process. Only three of the 40 interviews were judged to have a satisfactory termination to the interaction between mother and midwife. Privacy was also sadly lacking in nearly half the interviews, some of which were disturbed by interruptions on up to three occasions. This visibly affected the flow of conversation and reduced the sense of trust placed by the mother in the interviewing midwife (Methven 1982b, 1989).

☐ Communication and the booking interview

Communication skills have only recently been introduced into the midwifery training curriculum by the English National Board. Methven (1989) found that in every interview observed, the majority of questions used were closed in nature, confirming the conclusion of MacLeod Clark (1981) that 'consistent or habitual use of closed questions produces a powerful influence which will control or block development of a conversation'. Leading questions, generally considered to be a poor form of speech because they bias the answer received, also featured prominently. Similarly, use of the fixed alternative question encouraged mothers to choose one of two options when in reality more were available to her. In the few instances where open questions were asked, or a non-directive approach employed, the effect was destroyed by inhibiting the mother's reply with another closed question or use of clichés.

Most of the midwives observed, used the antenatal notes as an interview schedule. 'Beginning at the top and working down to the bottom' is how one expressed it. Consequently, the booking interview complied with the image of 'a form-filling exercise' (Thomson 1980) rather than 'purposeful, goal directed conversation' (Marriner 1979).

☐ Computerisation of antenatal records

In view of the above, it is hardly surprising that obstetricians in particular, have expressed such interest in the computer as a medium for obtaining information from mothers. According to Broadhurst (1988), 'computers can improve the quality of midwifery care'. This position has been endorsed by a great deal of research carried out over a number of years, notably by Professor Lilford (Lilford & Chard 1981, 1984; Brownbridge *et al* 1988; Catanzarite & Jelovsek 1988).

Smith (1984) describes how computers record a mother's history in her maternity unit. Computers are reported to be 'user friendly and midwifery oriented' (Broadhurst 1988), but it is suggested that while they may be an effective method of obtaining the data required from a mother and making legible records, they do not adequately meet the requirement of establishing a relationship with a mother, answering any questions she may have or supplying her with needed information about the rest of her pregnancy care. It is sobering to reflect that yet another traditionally acknowledged part of the midwives' role (CMB 1978) is likely to be eroded by modern technology, unless midwives can quickly demonstrate improved quality of outcome and increased consumer satisfaction with their conduct of the antenatal booking interview in order to reverse this trend.

☐ **Personally held case notes**

Another development which affects the antenatal booking interview is the opportunity for mothers to be responsible for their own obstetric records. The success of this venture is attested by many units (see Elbourne *et al* 1987; Elbourne & Lovell 1987; Lovell *et al* 1987). Wilton (1983) describes how the system works at Bradford.

Having personal access to her own records ensures that what is written about a mother must be acceptable to her. Parents are also more likely to question the meaning of statements made and to challenge the management of midwifery and obstetric care. This, more than any other factor, encourages personal accountability on the part of the interviewing midwife and a working partnership between parents and professionals in the management of pregnancy care. These factors must, in turn, affect the way in which the booking interview is approached and undertaken.

■ New initiatives in antenatal booking and care

An holistic approach to care of the mother can sometimes lead to intrusive questioning by an inexperienced interviewer (Methven 1982b). Some of this difficulty can be overcome if the interview is conducted in the mother's own home surroundings (ARM 1986, RCM 1987). It should then be possible to observe much about family relations, as well as the type and condition of facilities available in the home, without asking too many searching questions. Another advantage of recording the mother's history in her own home, is that she is usually more relaxed, and may have access to dates or other information required by the midwife which she would not have thought to bring with her to the hospital. Lasting relationships are also readily formed in this environment.

New initiatives in antenatal care, where the care is undertaken away from the main district general hospital, also facilitate increased freedom when obtaining a booking history. Thompson (1983), Penny (1986) and Taylor (1986) discuss the merits of day care, satellite and peripheral clinics respectively. The success of the Sighthill scheme is now well known (Staines 1983). Any system which promotes continuity of care for the mother or facilitates increased contact between her and one or a small group of midwives must ultimately be beneficial, whatever system of care and record keeping is employed. There is also evidence to suggest that these initiatives provide one way of overcoming the well publicised consumer complaints concerning waiting time in the clinic (Scott 1987). Methven (1982b) calculated that over two thirds of the total length of each booking visit was spent waiting in the clinic.

☐ **Continuity of care**

Where continuity of caregiver cannot be achieved, continuity of care by means of a care plan utilising individualised care (Heath *et al* 1986), or the midwifery process (Whitfield 1983), can be employed. By this means, some of the duplication of tasks and overlapping of roles reported by Robinson *et al* (1983) can be overcome.

A model specific to midwifery based on the philosophy of care operating within a maternity hospital, and its antenatal clinic in particular, can do much to determine not only the quality of midwifery care given to the mother, but also help to integrate the midwives involved into a coherent and effective team. A relationship initiated with a mother and the records established during the antenatal booking interview provide the obvious starting point for this.

It is not being suggested that midwives work in isolation from their obstetric colleagues, which would be detrimental to the welfare of both the mother and the fetus. Rather, midwives should be encouraged to be aware of the defined limits of their role, and feel confident to exercise rightful authority within it (Methven 1982b), while at the same time working in a complementary manner with colleagues who should acknowledge the midwife's statutory sphere of practice (UKCC 1989).

■ **The importance of the antenatal booking interview**

The antenatal booking interview is considered to be the most important aspect of midwifery care undertaken. It is the vehicle through which the essential relationship between mother and midwife is developed. It lays the foundation for the type and quality of midwifery care which the mother will receive and determines the extent to which parents can participate in decisions concerning the management of that care.

The booking interview opens the case notes which will become a permanent record of the mother's progress and the development of her baby, upon which subsequent research may be based. It should be viewed as much more than an information gathering exercise, even if this is widened to include a complete physical examination and certain investigations undertaken by the midwife. Partnership in care demands that the wishes of parents be ascertained and their views be incorporated into the records and reflected in the care planned for them during pregnancy, labour and the postnatal period.

The antenatal booking interview can provide a forum for dialogue, information giving and an opportunity to initiate parentcraft education where this is appropriate. If a mother is likely to be a poor attender at subsequent follow-up antenatal clinics, this visit may be strategic in affecting the future outcome of her pregnancy. The booking interview should therefore be regarded as the key element in midwifery care and the emphasis of midwifery education and the organisation of the maternity services should reflect this.

■ Recommendations for clinical practice in the light of currently available evidence

1. Several of the studies referred to in the above section, (notably Methven 1982b; Fawdry & Mutch 1986), indicate the need for further research to be undertaken. The necessity for a model of care specific to midwifery practice has been identified (Methven 1986b). There is also an obligation to establish exactly what information is required from a mother in order to plan midwifery care in partnership with her.

2. It has been demonstrated that the layout of antenatal records influences the type of information obtained from the mother, as well as the order and way in which the questions are asked (Methven 1982a). It is imperative, therefore, that midwives form part of every working party that is established to design maternity records or the content of computer programmes for use in obstetrics. Only in this way will the needs of parents and essential aspects of midwifery care be certain to be incorporated in the resulting documents and computer software.

3. Where this is not possible or there is no opportunity to modify existing records, ways of developing midwifery records that allow the mother to be considered from a holistic point of view and cared for as an individual should be considered. Planned care which can subsequently be evaluated against previously determined goals, has strong research backing (see, for example, Roper, Logan & Tierney 1982).

4. There is abundant evidence to support the case for the mother's records being kept by her (Wilton 1983; Elbourne *et al* 1987; Elbourne & Lovell 1987).

5. Imaginative ways of interviewing the mother in her home surroundings and increased integration of the midwifery service in order to foster improved continuity of care for the mother and her family should be further explored.

6. There is also scope for a reassessment of the purpose and function of the antenatal booking interview and permanent antenatal clinic staff could consider developing a philosophy of care relating to this. New staff working in the clinic could then be made aware of the aims and objectives for this initial interaction between mother and midwife as perceived by each maternity unit.

7. Some re-allocation of staff within the clinic has been suggested (Methven 1982b) so that midwives working there permanently should interview mothers, in order that relationships developed during this time can be maintained during pregnancy.

8. The booking interview should be considered as a task of high importance and not one of low status. Privacy for the interview should be fostered and interruptions banned while it is in progress.

9. It is recommended that student midwives should not undertake the unsupervised conduct of a booking interview until the final part of their training (Methven 1989). New methods of teaching communication skills and interview techniques should be explored for all midwives as well as those still in training.

10. It would appear to be necessary for midwives in each health authority to have clear guidance concerning the normal boundary of their sphere of practice in order that they may be certain about the type and range of decisions that can be taken by them. Similarly, midwives need to ensure that any locally agreed policies, procedures or protocols which already exist or may subsequently be developed are such that they allow the midwife to exercise professional judgement and to be accountable for her practice within these limits (UKCC 1989).

■ Practice check

1. *Ask permission to 'sit in' on the interaction between a midwife and a mother while her booking history is being recorded. Alternatively, you could watch a video recording of a booking interview, if this is available.*

● Observe the non-verbal communication that emanates from both mother and midwife during the interview, by noting eye contact, facial expression, posture, gestures or bodily movements, and any verbal para-language, such as grunts, laughter or other sounds which do not make ordinary words.

- On the basis of this information, what can be learnt about the individuals being observed and the relationship which develops between them during the interview?

2. *Obtain a tape recording of the conversation between a midwife and a mother during the booking interview.*

- Identify the categories of questions used by the midwife. Were these questions used appropriately?

- What kind of responses did these questions elicit from the mother? Would different questions have evoked different responses, and if so why?

- What alternative phrasing of questions could have been used?

- Were any leading questions used? Do you feel that these did influence the answer provided by the mother?

- Were there any instances of fixed alternative questions being used, which forced the mother to choose between two options when in reality there were more choices available to her?

- Overall, did the midwife tend to employ closed or direct questions or did she use open questions and a non-directive approach?

- In the light of the rest of this chapter how would you rate this interview?

3. *Observe another booking interview but this time concentrate on the interview technique employed by the midwife.*

- Does the midwife introduce herself to the mother? What information does she give to the mother about herself?

- How does the midwife address the mother? Is this appropriate?

- Can you identify any attempt by the midwife to develop a rapport with the mother?

- Is there any introduction or explanation about the purpose and function of the interview or does the midwife go straight ahead and start to obtain information from the mother?

- How does the midwife obtain the information she requires?

- Would you say the midwife was controlling the interview or is there a more balanced exchange between the interviewer and the respondent?

- Does the midwife use language appropriate for the particular mother being interviewed? Do you consider any unprofessional terminology is used? Are any terms used which the mother may not understand and which the midwife does not explain to her?

- Does the midwife use any probing questions to explore some areas more deeply?

- Are any techniques employed by the midwife to encourage the mother to talk more freely or in order to develop the conversation further?

- Does the midwife impart any information or is the interaction simply a fact finding exercise?

- Is the mother given any opportunity to ask questions?

- How does the midwife handle any questions raised by the mother?

- In what way does the midwife draw the interview to a close?

- How would you rate this interaction in the light of ideas presented in the rest of this chapter?

- Would you have handled the same situation any differently if you had been the interviewing midwife, and if so, how and why?

4. *Obtain the maternity case-notes from one of the mothers whose interview you have observed or listened to on tape. Compare what is written on the notes with the conversation you heard.*

- Do the notes adequately reflect the interaction which took place?

- Was anything said by mother or midwife which is not adequately recorded on the notes? If this is the case, why might this be?

- Is there sufficient information for another midwife who was not present at the interview to get to know the mother and her family as people from the records alone?

- How effectively could you make a plan for this mother's midwifery care during pregnancy and childbirth from the data available in these case-notes?

5. *Undertake a booking interview yourself in the manner in which it is usually conducted in your health authority. Ask permission from the mother for this to be recorded on tape, or video if this is available.*

- Observe the same features that you have looked at in the previous interviews undertaken by other midwives.

- Compare what you have recorded in the case-notes with the conversation that took place. Does it give an accurate reflection of the interaction?

- How do you rate your own interview performance? In what ways could it be improved?

6. *Using whatever means are available, identify all the information that you consider would be useful to obtain from a mother in order to plan her midwifery care. Justify your reason for each item.*

- Construct a framework (or interview schedule) which can be used as a guideline which will incorporate all these items.

- Ask permission to undertake your ideal booking interview with a mother, using the guideline you have designed.

- From the information thus obtained, identify the mother's needs and any problems which can be met by midwifery care.

- Design a plan of care for the mother you have interviewed.

- Indicate the aims of care and the way in which these goals might be achieved by a midwife.

- Indicate how, when and by whom the mother's care could be evaluated.

7. *Ask permission from a mother to try out two different approaches to conducting a booking interview.*
Begin with the traditional approach usually employed in your health authority. Then repeat the interview using the framework you have devised above or one based on a recognised model of nursing or midwifery care. Try as far as possible to use closed questions in the first interview and open or non-directive questions in the second.

- Compare the quality and quantity of information obtained from each interview.

- Which interview yielded the most suitable information to enable you to design a plan of midwifery care for that mother?

- Which interview did you feel more comfortable with? Why might this be?

- Ask a colleague who was not present for the interview to assess the recorded information and to plan care for the mother whom you interviewed using the data you have recorded.

- Which set of notes makes the mother 'come alive' as a person to your colleague?

- If your colleague was to be responsible for the future care of this mother which set of records and information would she find most helpful and why?

☐ **Acknowledgement**

The research which forms the basis of this chapter, in part fulfilment of an MSc in Nursing at the University of Manchester, was funded by a DHSS Research Student Grant, for which grateful acknowledgement is made.

■ References

Association of Radical Midwives 1986 The vision: proposals for the future of the maternity services. ARM, Ormskirk

Broadhurst M 1988 Computers can improve the quality of care. News item. Nursing Times 84 (48): 7

Brownbridge B, Lilford R, Tymbal Biscoe S 1988 Use of a computer to take booking histories in a hospital ante-natal clinic: acceptability to midwives, and patients and effects of the midwife-patient interaction. Medical Care 26: 474–87

Bryar R 1988 Midwifery and models of care. Midwifery 4 (3): 111–17

Catanzarite C, Jelovsek F K 1988 Computer applications in obstetrics. American Journal of Obstetricts and Gynaecology 156 (5): 1049–53

Chng P K, Hall M H, MacGillivery I 1980 An audit of ante-natal care: the value of the first ante-natal visit. British Medical Journal 281: 1184–86

Central Midwives Board 1978 Notices concerning a Midwife's Code of Practice. CMB, London

Crichton M 1989 Assessment of Needs Model. Manchester, awaiting publication

Crook I L 1988 Birth plans. The Journal of Family Medicine 13 (5): 116–21

Ekeocha C E O, Jackson P 1985 The birth plan experience. British Journal of Obstetrics and Gynaecology 92: 97–101

Elbourne D, Lovell A 1987 Holding the baby and your notes. The Health Service Journal 19 (3): 335

Elbourne D, Richardson M, Chalmers I, Waterhouse I, Holt E 1987 The Newbury maternity care study: a randomised controlled trial to assess a policy of women holding their own obstetric records. British Journal of Obstetrics and Gynaecology 94: 612–19

Fawdry R D S, Mutch M M 1986 Ante-natal history taking: what are we asking? Journal of Obstetrics and Gynaecology 5: 201–5. Reproduced in MIDIRS Information Pack No 3, Pregnancy and ante-natal care, December 1986

Green C 1985 The importance of the history and philosophy of science to the nursing process and professional development. Nurse Education Today 5 (4): 171–77

Heath J, Law G, Bradshaw J, Whitfield S 1986 Planned individualised care of the mother, baby and family unit. ENB Learning Resources Centre, Sheffield

Hope M 1983 Care cards. Midwives Chronicle 96 (1, 150; Supplement): 5–6

Hughes D F J, Goldstone L A 1989 Frameworks for midwifery care in Great Britain: an exploration into quality assurance. Midwifery 5 (4): 163–72

Julia N de 1980 The nursing interview. Australian Nursing Journal   10 (5): 38–9
Lilford R J 1987 Comparisons between written and computerised patient histories. British Medical Journal   289: 295–305
Lilford R J, Chard T 1981 Microcomputers in ante-natal care: a feasibility study on the booking interview. British Medical Journal   283: 533–6
Lilford R J, Chard T 1984 Computers in ante-natal care. In Chamberlain G (ed) Contemporary obstetrics. Butterworths, London
Lovell A, Zander L, James C, Foot S, Swan A, Reynolds A 1987 The St Thomas's Hospital maternity case notes study: a randomised controlled trial to assess the effects of giving mothers their own maternity case notes. Paediatric and Perinatal Epidemiology   1: 57–86
Macintyre S 1978 Some notes on record taking and making in the ante-natal clinic. Sociological Review   26 (3): 595–611
MacLeod Clark J 1981 Communication in nursing. Nursing Times   77 (1): 12–18
Maguire P, Rutter D 1976 Training medical students to communicate. In Bennett A C (ed) Communication between doctors and patients. National Provincial Hospitals Trust, Oxford University Press
Marriner A 1979 The nursing process: a scientific approach to nursing care. (2nd ed), Mosby, St Louis
Mayes G E 1987 Developing a model of care in Waltham Forest. Midwives Chronicle   100 (1, 198): v–ix
McFarlane J K, Castledine G 1982 A Guide to the practice of nursing using nursing process. Mosby, St Louis
Methven R C 1982a Recording an obstetric history or relating to a mother to be? Paper given at the Research and the Midwife Conferences, London and Glasgow
Methven R C 1982b An examination of the process and content of the ante-natal booking interview. Unpublished MSc thesis, University of Manchester
Methven R C 1986a Care plan for a woman having ante-natal care based on Orem's Self Care Model. In Webb C (ed) Woman's Health: midwifery and gynaecology. Hodder & Stoughton, Sevenoaks
Methven R C 1986b Care plan for a woman during pregnancy, labour and the puerperium, based on Henderson's Activities of Daily Living. In Webb C (ed) Woman's health: midwifery and gynaecology. Hodder & Stoughton, Sevenoaks
Methven R C 1989 Recording an obstetric history or relating to a pregnant woman? A study of the ante-natal booking interview. In Robinson S, Thomson A Midwives, research and childbirth Vol 1. Chapman & Hall, London
Midgley C 1988 Survey of use of models for nursing in midwifery. Unpublished BEd dissertation, Huddersfield Polytechnic
Oakley A 1983 The development of ante-natal care in the last eighty years. Maternal and Child Health   8 (2): 66–71
Open University 1979 Data Collection Procedures in Research Methods in Education and the Social Sciences. Block 4, DE 304. Open University Press, Milton Keynes
Orem D 1980 Nursing, concepts of practice (2nd ed) McGraw Hill, New York
Penny Y 1986 Mother's day. Nursing Times   9 (4): 37–8
Royal College of Midwives 1987 Report on the role and education of the midwife in the United Kingdom. RCM, London

Robinson S, Golden J, Bradley J 1983 A study of the role and responsibilities of the midwife. NERU Report No 1. Chelsea College, London University

Roper N, Logan W, Tierney A 1982 The elements of nursing (2nd ed). Churchill Livingstone, Edinburgh

Savage W 1980 Antenatal care: have Dr Ballantyne's aims been achieved? Midwife, Health Visitor and Community Nurse, Part 1 16 (5): 190–91; Part 2 16 (6): 238–42

Scott R M 1987 Waiting time in ante-natal booking clinics. Midwives Chronicle 100 (1, 196: 286–87)

Smith G 1984 A computer fit for kings. Midwifery Forum, Nursing Mirror 158 (14): iv–vi

Smith V M, Bass T A 1982 Communication for the health care team. Adapted for the UK by Faulkner A. Harper & Row, London

Staines C 1983 Moving forward in ante-natal care: the Sighthill Project, Edinburgh. Midwives Chronicle 96 (1, 147): Supplement 6–8

Symonds M 1980 Care of the pregnant mother. Midwife, Health Visitor and Community Nurse 16 (3): 94–9

Taylor R 1986 Satellite clinics in maternity care. Midwife, Health Visitor and Community Nurse 22 (8): 6–8

Thomson A M 1980 Planned or unplanned: are midwives ready for the 1980s? Midwives Chronicle 93 (1, 106) 68–72

Thompson J M 1983 Peripheral clinics. Midwives Chronicle 96 (1, 150): Supplement: 9–11

Towler J, Bramall J 1986 Midwives in history and society. Croom Helm, London

Walker J 1976 Midwife or obstetric nurse: some perceptions of the midwife and obstetrician on the role of the midwife. Journal of Advanced Nursing 1: 129–38

Whitfield S 1983 The midwifery process in practice. Midwives Chronicle 96 (1, 145): 186–9

Wilson J 1988 Individualised family care. Nursing Times 84 (16): 50–1

Wilton S 1983 Personally held case notes. Midwives Chronicle 96 (1, 150) Supplement: 7–8

United Kingdom Central Council for Nursing, Midwifery and Health Visiting 1989 A midwife's code of practice for midwives practising in the United Kingdom. UKCC, London

■ Suggested further reading

Breen D 1981 Talking with mothers. Jill Norman, London

Enkin M, Chalmers I 1982 Effectiveness and satisfaction in antenatal care. Spastics International Medical Publications Heinemann, London

Flint C, Poulengeris P 1987 The 'Know your midwife' report. Privately printed; available from 49 Peckarmans Wood, Syndenham Hill, London SE26 6RZ

Hall M, Macintyre S, Porter M 1985 Ante-natal care assessed. Aberdeen University Press, Aberdeen

Wright S 1986 Building and using a model of nursing. Edward Arnold, London

Chapter 4

Antenatal preparation of the breasts for breastfeeding

Jo Alexander

The desirability of encouraging a women to consider breastfeeding is widely acknowledged (Canadian Department of Health and Welfare 1979; Department of Health and Social Security 1988) but the need for physical preparation in pregnancy is an area for dispute (Hytten & Baird 1958; Inch 1987). Chalmers and Enkin (1982) believe 'that it is counterproductive to utilise practices or techniques which have not been demonstrated to be of benefit, yet which are time-consuming, sometimes uncomfortable and which place undue emphasis on physical ritual'. Midwives should therefore ensure that, whenever possible, the advice which they give is based upon sound research evidence.

In this chapter we discuss antenatal preparation such as the use of breast expression and massage; nipple rolling, rubbing, oral stimulation and the application of cream; testing for nipple inversion and non-protractility and the use of breast shells and Hoffman's exercises. The aim of the chapter is to describe the studies which have been conducted and to assist midwives to use their own clinical knowledge to decide on the validity of the research. It may also help them to plan their own trial.

■ It is assumed that you are already aware of the following:

- The anatomy of the breast and the physiology of lactation;
- The instructions which manufacturers include with breast shells designed for antenatal use.

■ Manual expression of colostrum

Waller (1946) was the first person to popularise the antenatal expression of colostrum. He believed that postnatal engorgement resulted in both sore nipples and a diminished milk supply and that it should therefore be relieved by expression. He wished women to acquire this skill antenatally so that they could treat engorgement quickly should it arise after delivery. In order to study the effect of this teaching, Waller alternately allocated 200 nulliparous women either to an experimental group or to a control. Those in the experimental group were taught breast massage and expression during the last three months of pregnancy, but women in both groups were given shells if their nipple protractility was thought to be deficient. At a superficial glance the intervention appears to have been very successful; those in the experimental group produced more milk throughout the first thirteen days, were considered to have less engorgement and nipple injury and were more likely to be breastfeeding on transfer home and at both three and six months postnatally. Several factors however (highlighted by Chalmers & Enkin 1982 and Inch 1989) make it impossible to interpret the significance of the antenatal intervention. The postnatal management of all the breastfeeding women within the hospital at this time involved the limitation of suckling time, a practice which is thought likely to increase engorgement (RCM 1988). Expression after feeds was used for all women who became engorged and some were also given stilboestrol; we are not told how many women in each arm of the trial required these treatments. The fact that the postnatal care differed so extensively from current midwifery practice makes it impossible to draw firm conclusions from this study. Chalmers and Enkin (1982) also indicated that the experimental group received additional attention from a midwife both antenatally and postnatally, and other researchers (Housten *et al* 1981) have demonstrated that even additional non-interventionist midwifery support enhances breastfeeding success.

Blaikley *et al* (1953) replicated Waller's study allocating 183 women to the control and 181 to the experimental group, the latter being taught to carry out breast massage and colostrum expression for the last four to eight weeks of pregnancy. The postnatal management of all the women delivered in hospital involved manual expression after each feed for at least the first seven days and also between feeds if the breasts were filling very rapidly. Stilboestrol was prescribed for 'overfilling'. Of the women delivered in hospital those in the experimental group were significantly more likely to be breastfeeding six months postnatally than the controls, but this difference was not shown by those in the experimental group who delivered at home. The researchers therefore concluded that it was the supervision in the postnatal period which mattered and that the antenatal management served only as a preparation for this. They stressed that they considered the value to be in 'learning expression for use at the lying-in rather than expression to ensure patency of the milk ducts.' The criticisms levelled at Waller's study (1946) are also relevant to the paper by Blaikley *et al* and thus again it is not possible to interpret the significance of the antenatal intervention.

Whitley (1978) carried out a retrospective study of 34 women one year after they had completed their antenatal classes. The sample consisted of primiparous and multiparous women who had a telephone interview lasting up to three-quarters of an hour. Some women had carried out antenatal breast expression and some nipple rolling, some had done both and others nothing at all. It appeared that expression made no difference to the incidence of engorgement and those who had expressed, breastfed on average for a shorter period of time than those who had not. This is perhaps surprising as one would have expected them to be the more motivated group having chosen to expend so much time on their antenatal preparation. Some professionals would also have expected their added familiarity with handling their breasts to be to their advantage. It appeared that antenatal nipple rolling did not prevent sore nipples (of the 24 women who had carried out this preparation 16 had soreness; of the 10 women who had not, 5 had this problem).

In 1983 Mundy reported having asked 66 primiparae during their post-natal stay in hospital whether they had carried out antenatal expression. Nine replied that they had and 57 that they had not. By the sixth postnatal day, seven of the babies whose mothers had expressed had gained weight as opposed to 50 of the babies in the other group. At the end of the first month, all those who had expressed were still breastfeeding as compared to 83 per cent of those who had not; this is perhaps not surprising as the women who had chosen to express antenatally were presumably an especially highly motivated group. By nine months one of the group who had expressed antenatally had had mastitis, as had two of the group who had not. This study has many problems. Apart from its small size, it is also difficult to know how accurately the women reported their antenatal preparation. When asked by a midwife on a postnatal ward whether she had expressed her breasts antenatally, a mother might feel tempted to answer yes even if the attempt had been at best half-hearted. It is however true that other studies have also suggested the possibility of a link between antenatal expression and mastitis. This study cannot be used to argue in favour of antenatal expression.

Ingleman-Sundberg (1958) describes a trial in which he taught 313 women to begin breast massage and colostrum expression from 20 weeks. The two other consultants gave the 343 women under their care no such instruction. This is not an ideal way to create a control group but the researcher states that the mothers whom the three consultants generally cared for had the same distribution for social group, age and parity (no figures are given to support this). During their postnatal stay in hospital the mothers in both groups were cared for by the same 'nurses' and carried out manual expression after every feed. There was no significant difference between the two groups in the percentage who were fully breastfeeding on transfer home nor in the total amount of milk produced on the seventh day (the latter was calculated by test weighing and adding the volume expressed after each feed). However the frequency of mastitis during the postnatal hospital stay (the average being eight to ten days) was 0.88 per cent plus or minus 0.51 for the controls and 2.88 per cent plus or minus 0.95 for the intervention group. This is just short of statistical significance ($p < 0.06$). Ingleman-Sundberg recommends that the technique should only be carried out antenatally by those with poor nipple protractility but does not explain why it should benefit even this group.

Brown and Hurlock (1975) designed a trial with what they considered to be a perfect control group. Fifty-seven women with no previous breast feeding experience each carried out antenatal preparation of one breast only, the breast to be prepared being determined by the toss of a coin. The women were randomly allocated to carry out either nipple rolling, colostrum expression or to apply Masse ® cream twice daily from 37 weeks. Postnatally nipple damage was rated for the first 10 days, daily whilst in hospital and then on alternate days. The observers were blind both to the treatment allocation and to which breast had been prepared. The mother completed a questionnaire after every feed which included rating the sensitivity of each nipple on a four point scale; (the value of these subjective ratings is discussed on page 62). The nipples prepared by expression or Masse ® cream application did not differ significantly from the unprepared nipple on either the objective or subjective assessments. Those prepared by rolling gave rise to slightly less damage and pain than their unprepared counterparts. Chalmers and Enkin (1982) report that 'this difference was considered by the authors to be too small to be clinically significant and was also of borderline statistical significance ($p = 0.05$)'. There was no significant difference between the three active methods of preparation. Atkinson (1979) has however pointed out that the time available for treatment was very short.

The babies of mothers who had expressed one breast antenatally did not gain more weight than the other babies and the researchers concluded that it is therefore unlikely that this intervention increases milk flow. The only other measure on which the groups differed was the average length of time between feeds, this being longer for the nipple rolling group; it is difficult to think why. The researchers state that light-haired, fair-skinned women did not appear to have more difficulty with nipple damage, a finding that is also supported by Brockway (1986) but this latter study needs to be treated with caution.

Brown and Hurlock (1975) state that the women who reported having failed to carry out their antenatal preparations were excluded from the analysis. As the researchers themselves both taught the preparation and subsequently asked about compliance, it is possible that women who had not done what they were asked may have found it difficult to give an honest reply. It would therefore have been better to analyse the results simply on the basis of the allocated treatment group rather than to have made these exclusions; that is to have analysed by 'intention to treat'. It is also unfortunate that women who remained in hospital for longer than the average postnatal stay were discarded from the sample as presumably feeding difficulty may have been one of the reasons why they stayed. The paper presents very little numerical data but gives the results of statistical tests. Unfortunately neither Brown and Hurlock (1975) nor Ingleman-Sundberg (1958) measured breastfeeding rates after discharge from hospital.

■ Toughening of the nipple epithelium

A recent survey (Martin & White 1988) of 8154 births in Great Britain found that 28 per cent of breastfeeding women who had problems with their feeding whilst in hospital had sore or cracked nipples and 27 per cent of women who stopped breastfeeding within two weeks of delivery gave painful breasts or nipples as one of their reasons for discontinuing. This common occurrence of nipple soreness and its adverse effect on the duration of feeding has led to considerable interest in its prevention. Margaret Mead (cited in Newton 1952) apparently observed a much lower incidence of nipple soreness amongst breastfeeding women of 'primitive' cultures than amongst those of industrialised societies and popularly this has been ascribed to the toughening of the nipple epithelium by exposure to abrasion, temperature change and sunlight (Walker 1987; Inch 1989). Many different antenatal treatments have been suggested to toughen nipples but comparatively little attempt has been made to investigate their efficacy.

Atkinson (1979) enrolled 22 right-handed primigravidae with protractile nipples to prepare one nipple from 34 weeks gestation. The side to be prepared was assigned alternately. Preparation consisted of a combination of gentle rubbing with a terry towel for about 15 seconds daily, nipple rolling twice daily (taking the nipple between the thumb and forefinger and pulling it out firmly, then rolling it between the fingers for two minutes) and leaving the bra flap down for two hours a day to allow the outer clothes to rub against the nipple. The 'control side' was given only a daily wash with water. For the first five days postnatally the mother rated the sensitivity of each nipple on completion of every feed, using a sliding scale ranging from 'no pain' to 'extreme pain'. Suckling time was restricted throughout this time and both breasts were used at each feed. Seventeen women completed the study. Atkinson found that there was significantly less overall pain in the conditioned group ($p = 0.01$) and, in particular, less extreme pain ($p = 0.01$). Six women however reported no difference and it must be remembered that the study was very small. The author herself comments that the mothers may have been biased depending on whether they believed the preparation to be effective and also by virtue of the considerable amount of time which they had given to it. This criticism could also be made in relation to the subjective ratings in Brown and Hurlock's study (1975) but unlike Atkinson they also included ratings of nipple damage made by a 'blind' observer. Atkinson recorded that for their unprepared nipple, the seven fair skinned women reported significant pain more often than the seven average-complexioned women, the three women with olive skins reporting the least; this is in contrast with the findings of Brown and Hurlock in their larger study of 57 women.

Fleming (1984) carried out a partial replication of Atkinson's study recruiting the 17 women who completed her trial from childbirth classes. An identical schedule of antenatal preparation was carried out and the same rating scale of nipple sensitivity was used by the mothers throughout their hospital stay; (feeds involving one breast only, or those for which a nipple shield was used were excluded). The conditioned nipples were significantly more likely ($p < 0.025$) to give rise to no pain at all or only slight soreness than the unconditioned nipples, they were also significantly less likely to cause extreme pain ($p < 0.01$). Five women however reported no difference between their conditioned and unconditioned sides. Unfortunately it is not possible to draw conclusions about the efficacy of the antenatal interventions from this study either, both because Atkinson's comments about the possibly biased nature of the mothers' ratings of nipple sensitivity still apply and because of the very small sample size.

Another study to which Atkinson's comments are also relevant is that described by Storr (1988). The 25 primigravidae who had carried out twice daily treatment of one of their nipples from 34 weeks (rubbing with a terry towel and rolling the nipple), reported significantly less overall pain on the experimental side ($p = 0.001$). The validity of this finding is further called into question by the fact that we are not told whether the women chose which breast to prepare or whether this was alternately allocated. If left to their own choice it would seem likely that they would treat the side which they found easiest to handle and this would probably also be the side on which they would have less difficulty fixing the baby postnatally. The researcher in fact tells us that many of the women reported that nursing was easier on the experimental side. The study also included the massage of the experimental breast after each feed as a measure to reduce engorgement; even this on its own would make it difficult to interpret the significance of the antenatal intervention.

L'Esperance (1980) investigated 16 factors which were popularly believed to relate to nipple pain during early breastfeeding. One hundred and two women were interviewed within 24 hours of delivery and studied for the first four days. Two of the factors investigated were found to have significant negative associations with nipple pain. Limiting the duration of feeds was not associated with less discomfort and in fact short feeds were significantly more likely than long ones to be associated with pain. The researcher also claimed that women with poorly protractile nipples were significantly less likely ($p < 0.05$) to have moderate to extreme discomfort at 48 hours than those with protractile nipples. This latter finding must be treated with caution as the researcher herself suggests that, due to fixing difficulty, the mothers with poorly protractile nipples may have been feeding less frequently than the others. Also we are not told whether the assessment of nipple protractility was made before the first feed, but simply that it was made in the first 24 hours. Several authors (Waller 1946; Hytten & Baird 1958; Gunther 1973; Otte 1975; Helsing 1984) suggest that a baby with a vigorous suck can improve anatomically poor nipples. It is therefore possible that some women with nipples which were 'poor' at the time of delivery were protractile by the time of examination as several feeds may have taken place and Otte (1975) suggests that nipples which are 'corrected' by vigorous sucking are at especial risk of persistent soreness and cracking. For these reasons this aspect of her study needs to be treated with caution.

The only factor which L'Esperance found to have a significant positive correlation with nipple pain was engorgement. The 13 other factors investigated included previous breastfeeding experience, skin sensitivity and antenatal conditioning from clothing or lovemaking and none was found to have a significant relationship with nipple pain. As with the remaining four studies described below, the mothers were asked retrospectively about their antenatal breast preparation and therefore the findings in respect of this are unfortunately of anecdotal interest only.

Nicholson (1985) studied 1902 breastfeeding women, the main purpose of her trial being to assess three methods of treating cracked nipples. She asked them retrospectively whether they had carried out any form of antenatal nipple preparation and found that those who had were more likely to develop cracks than those who had not, but that this difference did not reach statistical significance.

It also appears that Clark (1985) retrospectively asked the 114 mothers involved in her trial whether they had carried out antenatal preparation (the main purpose of her study was to compare four methods of postnatal nipple care). She states that on the fourth postnatal day those who had performed antenatal preparation were less likely to be tender than those who had not but more likely to have cracks. The nature of the antenatal preparation is not specified.

Jones (1984) in the report of her study of 649 breastfeeding women stated that postnatal problems did not seem to be reduced by the carrying out of antenatal preparation or the receipt of antenatal advice. Unfortunately she gave no evidence to support her statement.

Hewat and Ellis (1987) also questioned women retrospectively about their antenatal nipple preparation, some of their 23 subjects having carried out a variety of the following: nipple rolling, nipple rubbing, breast massage, application of a substance, going bra-less, and oral stimulation. They found that antenatal preparation (either educational or physical) had no significant relationship with nipple pain but that oral stimulation was correlated significantly ($p < 0.03$) with less postnatal nipple trauma. Seven women had experienced this practice and, despite the possibility that it might cause oxytocin release, none had delivered preterm. They too found there to be no significant relationship between nipple pain or trauma and hair or skin colour.

Thus none of the studies outlined above, nor those by Brown and Hurlock (1975) or Whitley (1978) as previously described, provide satisfactory evidence of any clinically significant advantage to be gained by the antenatal preparation of normally protractile nipples. Three studies (Newton 1952; Gans 1958; Riordan 1985) investigating the prophylactic application of various substances to nipples postnatally have also failed to demonstrate any beneficial effect and in some instances showed an increase in nipple pain (see Chapter 2 in Volume 3 for further details). This raises further doubt as to the efficacy of applying such substances to the nipples antenatally. Finally, it has to be said that if nipple 'toughening' did make a difference, one would expect women who had breastfed before to have considerably less postnatal soreness than those breastfeeding for the first time. Gunther (1945), L'Esperance (1980), Jones (1984), Nicholson (1985) and Martin and White (1988) all found that previous breastfeeding experience afforded no protection from such soreness.

■ Nipple protractility

Cineradiographic work (Ardran *et al* 1958) and ultrasound studies (Weber *et al* 1985; Woolridge 1986) have demonstrated that a breastfeeding baby forms a 'teat' from the nipple and surrounding breast tissue and that this 'teat' is about three times as long as the nipple at rest (this is further discussed in the chapter by Sally Inch, 'Postnatal care relating to breastfeeding' in the volume in this series on *Postnatal Care*). Subsequently the Royal College of Midwives (RCM 1988) has stated that the shape of the nipple is less important than the protractility of the underlying tissues as it is this which governs the ability of the baby to make an effective 'teat'. Evidence of the importance of protractility is provided by the work of Hytten and Baird (1958) who used quarter-inch diameter ball-ended callipers to compress the areola immediately behind the nipple and hence produce a quantitative measurement of protractility; the smaller the 'bite' size the greater the ability of the tissue to elongate. One hundred and seventy primiparous women were measured and of the 26 whose 'bite' size was 6 mm or more at delivery, nine had difficulty fixing their babies. Of the 144 whose 'bite' size was less than 6 mm, four had difficulty ($p < 0.001$).

A link between poor protractility and fixing difficulty, nipple damage, diminished milk production and lactation failure has been claimed by numerous authors (Waller 1946; Naish 1948; Hoffman 1953; Blaikley *et al* 1953; Gunther 1973; Walker 1987; Sweet 1988), some of them presenting supporting evidence. In contrast there are two reports which call into question the reported link with nipple damage. The apparent finding by L'Esperance (1980) that poor protraction had a protective effect against soreness has already been discussed. Secondly, Hytten (1954) in his study of 6456 women claimed that the incidence of soreness was no higher in those with poor protraction than in the rest. We are not told when nipple protractility was assessed postnatally and thus his finding needs to be treated with caution for the same reason as that of L'Esperance.

Less certain than the adverse effect of poor protractility on breastfeeding is the predictive value of antenatal nipple examination. Hytten (1954) reported that of the primigravidae who were found to have poor protractility in early pregnancy, 16 per cent had consequent breastfeeding difficulties as opposed to 3.5 per cent of those who had had normal protraction; (no antenatal treatment of poor protraction was advised). He concluded that whilst the antenatal examination did indeed have some predictive value, the majority of those who have poor protraction in early pregnancy will in fact have no consequent breastfeeding difficulties.

An additional question mark over the need for antenatal treatment of poor protractility is raised by Hytten and Baird (1958) who suggest that protractility spontaneously improves during pregnancy. They found that 34.7 per cent of the 170 primigravidae whom they examined in early pregnancy had poor protraction but that, without any treatment, this had fallen to 7.7 per cent by the first postnatal day. Their theory was further supported by finding a reduction in 'bite' size over this period of time. Despite this it must still be remembered that no evidence has yet been produced to indicate which nipples are likely to improve and therefore most writers agree on the need for antenatal examination and subsequent treatment of inversion or non-protractility (Waller 1939; Naish 1948; Nicholson 1985; Sweet 1988).

Hauden and Mahler (1983) describe an inverted nipple as being one which is situated on a plane below the areola. A non-protractile nipple is however less easy to define and the most widely advocated test is that described by Waller (1946): 'in imitation of the action of the baby's jaws the areola is pinched (between the tumb and forefinger) just beyond the nipple's base'. If this causes the nipple to project it is considered as satisfactory and classed as being protractile. He states that those which do not project or which retract are attached too firmly to the deep structures of the breast and are classed as non-protractile. Simple inspection of the nipple is not enough and it is perhaps more acceptable if the woman carries out the 'pinch' herself. Hytten and Baird (1958) stress that this 'pinch' test should be performed later rather than earlier in pregnancy so that treatment can be reserved for the small group whose nipples remain poorly protractile at this time.

The most widely described method of antenatal treatment is the use of shells. No controlled trial has yet been completed in which the outcome for women given shells during pregnancy is contrasted with that for a similar group of women who are not. Waller (1946) conducted a controlled trial to investigate the effect of antenatal expression on postnatal engorgement (this has been described earlier). Women from both the control and the experimental groups were given shells as necessary and he states that 'in all but the worst types of deformity the results are good' but gives no evidence for this claim. Blaikley *et al* (1953) replicated Waller's trial and thus also had no control group. Their conclusion that 'good improvement can be promised to nearly all cases ... if they wear [shells]' cannot therefore be considered valid. Hytten and Baird (1958) suggest that the small group of women in their study who failed to show spontaneous improvement of nipple protractility during pregnancy (see above), might constitute the group which Waller and Blaikley *et al* found resistant to treatment.

Antenatal manipulation is also used to treat inverted or nonprotractile nipples and Hoffman (1953) gives the most detailed description of the exercises designed to stretch the adhesions anchoring the nipple to the deeper structures of the breast. 'The procedure is one of placing the thumbs, or the forefingers, close to the inverted nipple, then pressing into the breast tissue quite firmly and gradually pushing the fingers away from the areola' and thus from each other. This is done five times in succession with the fingers first in a horizontal and then in a vertical position (Fig. 4.1). He recommends that the woman should then grasp the nipple at its base and ease it out a bit further.

There has as yet been no controlled trial of antenatal manipulation and authors differ in their opinion of its effectiveness. Hoffman (1953), Otte (1975), Dutton (1979) and Cadwell (1981) advocate its use while Naish (1948), Eastman (1950), Waller (1957), and James (1981) consider it ineffective. The author of this chapter is currently conducting a randomised controlled trial to evaluate the use of shells alone, Hoffman's exercises alone and shells with Hoffman's exercises in relation to a no-treatment group. (This trial is now being extended to other midwifery units and via the National Childbirth Trust.) Lawrence (1985) cautions that nipple stimulation may cause uterine contractions and is supported by the work of Jhirad and Vago (1973), Viegas *et al* (1984), and Frager and Miyazaki (1987). Alexander's data thus far however do not indicate that preterm delivery is any more common amongst women using Hoffman's exercises.

Several other methods of antenatal management such as metal and rubber nipple shields, surgical elevation and suction have been described (Naish 1948; Cotterman *et al* 1978; Gangal & Gangal 1978; Hauden & Mahler 1983; Lawrence 1985; Poole 1987). These methods are not widely practised, however, and in some cases would be unlikely to be generally acceptable.

The evidence relating to the prevalence of poor protractility is confusing. The lowest figure for nulliparous women examined in early pregnancy is the 14 per cent quoted by Hytten (1954); the highest in excess of 75.5 per cent (Waller 1946). The only study including multiparous women is that by

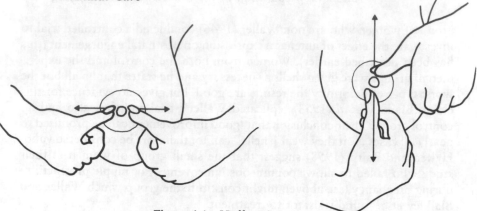

Figure 4.1 Hoffman's exercises

Hytten and Baird (1958) who found poor protractility in 10.7 per cent of the primiparous women examined in early pregnancy but in none of the 29 women examined whose parity was greater than one. In the same study they found the prevalence of nulliparae to be 34.7 per cent and therefore concluded that 'the changes in the nipple brought about by pregnancy seems to be cumulative'. It seems reasonable however to assume that they only examined the nipples of those intending to breastfeed and it is therefore possible that the observed lower prevalence figure in multiparous women is due, at least in part, to a decision by those with very poor protractility not to attempt to breastfeed after a previous failure; (the link between poor protractility and breastfeeding failure has been discussed above). It may also be relevant that details are not given as to whether the multiparous women examined had breastfed before. None of the studies indicate whether the women had a unilateral or a bilateral problem and it appears that occasionally nipples which were protractile in early pregnancy have ceased to be so by the first postnatal day (Hytten & Baird 1958).

In view of the current lack of evidence regarding the efficacy of shells and Hoffman's exercises, each clinician has to decide for him or herself whether to conduct the 'pinch test' antenatally and then to discuss treatment accordingly. What is certain however is that if the examination is carried out the results must be dealt with sensitively and the mother assured that non-protractility may well prove of little significance to a well-positioned baby who sucks vigorously (Otte 1975). If this is not done and the woman is simply led to believe that she may have difficulty breastfeeding 'this will only serve to damage her confidence and can be a self-fulfilling prophecy' (RCM 1988). It should also be remembered that women with inverted nipples may have had severe doubts since adolescence about their ability to breastfeed (Poole 1987) and the discussion following an antenatal examination could well be reassuring for them.

In 1944 the then Ministry of Health indicated that a distaste for breastfeeding might be engendered by the suggestion that an elaborate routine of antenatal preparation was necessary. 'We think it possible that with an anxious type of woman too much stress on preparation of the breasts may alarm and discourage her to such an extent that she will refuse to initiate breastfeeding' (Ministry of Health 1944). That the thought of antenatal preparation should sway some women against breastfeeding seems tragic and highlights the fine balance that the midwife has to achieve between the psychological and physical needs of her client.

■ Recommendations for clinical practice in the light of currently available evidence:

1. That the technique of breast expression should not be taught antenatally;

2. That nipple protractility should be assessed late in the second or early in the third trimester, the results being thoroughly discussed with the woman. If she is found to have an inverted or nonprotractile nipple she should then choose whether she wishes to have treatment and if so, what;

3. That no other preparation of the breasts or nipples is required;

4. That antenatally the ordinary daily wash of the nipples should not involve soap as it destroys the natural protective lubrication (Newton 1952);

5. That women should not be given the impression that it is essential to wear a bra. There is no evidence as to whether wearing a bra in pregnancy by day or by night conveys any physical benefit. This matter should simply be governed by the woman's wishes and comfort. If she wishes to wear one, it should be well-fitted and practical; further discussion of desirable design features should be sought elsewhere.

■ Practice check

● Consider the antenatal advice that you give, or that given within your unit, in the light of the evidence discussed in this chapter.

● Do you consider that non-protractility adversely affects breastfeeding? What data are you using to support your views?

● Observe how the length and shape of a nipple prior to a breastfeed compares with its length on completion.

- If you are unfamiliar with the 'pinch test' try to involve it in your clinical practice so that you can assess its use for yourself.

- Could you teach Hoffman's exercises?

- Have you tried wearing antenatal breast shells? Women may ask you about their convenience and comfort.

☐ **Acknowledgement**

I should like to acknowledge the assistance and encouragement received from Margaret Duckett, Margaret Gulson, Sally Inch and Mary Renfrew during the writing of this chapter.

■ **References**

Ardran G M, Kemp F H, Lind J 1958 A cineradiographic study of breastfeeding. British Journal of Radiology 31: 156–62

Atkinson L D 1979 Prenatal nipple conditioning for breastfeeding. Nursing Research 28(5): 267–71

Blaikley J, Clarke S, MacKeith R, Ogden K M 1953 Breastfeeding: factors affecting success. Journal of Obstetrics and Gynaecology of the British Empire 60: 657–69

Brockway L 1986 Hair colour and problems in breastfeeding. Midwives Chronicle 99: 1,178: 66–7

Brown M S, Hurlock J T 1975 Preparation of the breast for breastfeeding. Nursing Research 24(6): 448–51

Cadwell K 1981 Improving nipple graspability for success at breastfeeding. Journal of Obstetric, Gynecologic and Neonatal Nursing 10(4): 277–79

Canadian Department of Health & Welfare 1979 Breastfeeding: an awareness programme from Health & Welfare Canada and the Canadian Paediatric Society. Ministry of National Health & Welfare, Ottawa

Chalmers I, Enkin M 1982 Miscellaneous interventions in pregnancy: RH immunization; preparation for breastfeeding; external cephalic version. In Enkin M, Chalmers I (eds) Effectiveness and satisfaction in antenatal care. Spastics International Medical Publications; Heinemann, London

Clark M 1985 A study of four methods of nipple care offered to post partum mothers. The New Zealand Nursing Journal 78(6): 16–18

Cotterman J, Goodman N, Bradford R 1978 Breastfeeding (a letter). Journal of Obstetric, Gynecologic and Neonatal Nursing 7(6): 48–9

Department of Health and Social Security 1988 Present day practice in infant feeding: third report: 14. (Report on Health and Social Subjects 32). HMSO, London

Dutton M A 1979 A breastfeeding protocol. Journal of Obstetric, Gynecologic and Neonatal Nursing 8(3): 151–55

Eastman N J 1950 Williams' Obstetrics (10th ed): 971. Appleton-Century-Crofts, New York

Fleming P A 1984 The effect of prenatal nipple conditioning on postpartum nipple pain of breastfeeding women. Health Care for Women International 5(5): 453–57

Frager N B, Miyazaki F S 1987 Intrauterine monitoring of contractions during breast stimulation. Obstetrics and Gynecology 69(5): 767–69

Gangal H T, Gangal M H 1978 Suction method for correcting flat nipples or inverted nipples. Plastic and Reconstructive Surgery 61(2): 294–96

Gans B 1958 Breast and nipple pain in early stages of lactation. British Medical Journal ii: 830–32

Gunther M 1945 Sore nipples – causes and prevention. Lancet ii: 590–93

Gunther M 1973 Infant feeding. Penguin Books, Harmondsworth

Hauden D J, Mahler D 1983 A simple method for the correction of the inverted nipple. Plastic and Reconstructive Surgery 71(4): 556–59

Helsing E, Savage King F 1984 Preparing mothers for breastfeeding. The Nursing Journal of India 75(7): 155–56

Hewat R J, Ellis D J 1987 A comparison of the effectiveness of two methods of nipple care. Birth 14(1): 41–5

Hoffman J B 1953 A Suggested treatment for inverted nipples. American Journal of Obstetrics and Gynaecology 66(2): 346–48

Houston M J, Howie PW, Cook A, McNeilly A S 1981 Do breastfeeding mothers get the home support they need? Health Bulletin 39(3): 166–72

Hytten F E 1954 Clinical and chemical studies in human lactation IX: breastfeeding in hospital. British Medical Journal II (4902): 1447–52

Hytten F E, Baird D 1958 The development of the nipple in pregnancy. Lancet i (7032): 1201–04

Inch S 1987 Difficulties with breastfeeding: midwives in disarray? Journal of the Royal Society of Medicine 80: 53–7

Inch S 1989 Antenatal promotion of breastfeeding. In Enkin MW, Keirse M J N C, Chalmers I (eds) Effective care in pregnancy and childbirth. Oxford University Press, Oxford

Ingleman-Sundberg A, 1958 The value of antenatal massage of nipples and expression of colostrum. Journal of Obstetrics and Gynaecology of the British Empire 65: 448–49

James T 1981 Curiosa paedliatrica V: inverted nipples, South African Medical Journal 60(15): 598

Jhirad A, Vago T 1973 Induction of labour by breast stimulation. Obstetrics and Gynecology 41(3): 347–50

Jones D 1984 Breastfeeding problems. Nursing Times 80(33): 53–4

Lawrence R A 1985 Breastfeeding – a guide for the medical profession (2nd ed). Mosby, St Louis

L'Esperance C M 1980 Pain or pleasure: the dilemma of early breastfeeding. Birth and the Family Journal 7(1): 21–6

Martin J, White A 1988 Infant feeding 1985: 29, 34–5. HMSO, London

Ministry of Health 1944 The breastfeeding of infants – a report of the advisory committee on mothers and children. Public Health Medical Subjects Report No 91. Ministry of Health, London

Mundy D 1983 Summary of a survey on antenatal expression. Midwife Health Visitor and Community Nurse 20: 286–89

Naish F C 1948 Breastfeeding – a guide to the natural feeding of infants. Oxford University Press, London

Newton N 1952 Nipple pain and nipple damage – problems in the management of breastfeeding. Journal of Pediatrics 41: 411–23

Nicholson W 1985 Cracked nipples in breastfeeding mother – a randomised trial of three methods of management. Nursing Mothers Association of Australia 21(4): 7–10

Otte M J 1975 Correcting inverted nipples – an aid to breastfeeding. American Journal of Nursing 75(3): 454–56

Poole K 1987 A matter of confidence. New Generation 6(1): 33–4

Riordan J 1985 The effectiveness of topical agents in reducing nipple soreness of breastfeeding mothers. Journal of Human Lactation 1(3): 36–41

Royal College of Midwives 1988 Successful breastfeeding: 12,55 Holywell Press, Oxford

Storr G B 1988 Prevention of nipple tenderness and breast engorgement in the postpartal period. Journal of Obstetric, Gynecologic and Neonatal Nursing 17(3): 203–09

Sweet B R 1988 Mayes' midwifery: a textbook for midwives: 144–6. Baillière Tindall, London

Viegas O A C, Arulkumaran S, Gibb D M F, Ratnam S S 1984 Nipple stimulation in late pregnancy causing uterine hyperstimulation and profound fetal bradycardia. British Journal of Obstetrics and Gynaecology 91: 364–66

Walker M 1987 Letter. Birth 14(3): 159

Waller H 1939 Clinical studies in lactation. Heinemann, London

Waller H 1946 The early failure of breastfeeding: a clinical study of its causes and their prevention. Archives of Disease in Childhood 21: 1–12

Waller H K 1957 The breasts and breastfeeding: 14. Heinemann, London

Weber F, Woolridge M W, Baum J D 1985 An ultrasonographic analysis of sucking and swallowing in newborn infants. Developmental Medicine and Child Neurology 28: 19-24

Whitley N 1978 Preparation for breastfeeding: a one year follow up of 34 nursing mothers. Journal of Obstetric, Gynecologic and Neonatal Nursing 7(3): 44–8

Woolridge M W 1986 The anatomy of infant feeding. Midwifery 2: 164–71

■ Suggested further reading

Royal College of Midwives 1988 Successful Breastfeeding. Holywell Press, Oxford

Inch S 1989 Antenatal promotion of breastfeeding. In Enkin M W, Keirse M J N C, Chalmers I (eds) Effective care in pregnancy and childbirth. Oxford University Press, Oxford

Minchin M K 1985 Breastfeeding matters. Alma Publications; Allen & Unwin, Melbourne

Lawrence R A 1985 Breastfeeding – a guide for the medical profession (2nd ed). Mosby, St Louis

Samuel P 1985 Thinking about breastfeeding? National Childbirth Trust, London

Chapter 5

Maternal alcohol and tobacco use during pregnancy

Moira Plant

For centuries alcohol has been recommended for medicinal purposes by midwives, doctors and other health professionals. Indeed until quite recently alcohol was used in some places to treat premature labour (Lele 1982). To confuse the issue even more, it was also used to induce mid-trimester abortion (Gomel & Carpenter 1973). The scientific literature may be sparse but old wives' tales are numerous on this subject. The notion that the cure for unwanted pregnancy is 'a bottle of gin and a hot bath' is still heard in some areas. This prescription is more likely to cause acute alcohol poisoning, even death.

The profusion of roles attributed to alcohol is further compounded by the stereotype of the Sairey Gamp figure delivering the babies of the poor. Alcohol has been linked with pregnancy and the management of labour for centuries. It therefore becomes all the more important to assess this connection in a critical and scientific way.

■ **It is assumed you are already aware of the following:**

● The basic physiological effects of alcohol and tobacco;

● The literature available, either from local bodies or from national organisations such as the HEA, to recommend to clients who want advice on alcohol or tobacco use and/or its cessation;

● What specialist counselling services are available in your area for problem drinkers.

■ The effects of alcohol

The majority of people who consume light to moderate amounts of alcohol are unlikely to suffer ill effects related to their drinking. However there are times and situations when even small amounts of alcohol can cause problems. Drinking before driving is a major cause of accidents, injuries and fatalities. Drunken drivers kill over 1000 people each year in the UK alone.

Alcohol is a drug which, after ingestion, passes rapidly into the bloodstream. Most of it (over 90 per cent) is broken down by the liver, hence the connection between heavy drinking and liver disease. The remainder is excreted in sweat and urine. Each unit of alcohol (see Fig. 5.1, page 76) puts the blood alcohol level up by roughly 15 mg per 100 millilitres of blood. (The drinking driving limit is 80 mg per 100 ml of blood.) On average it takes one hour for each unit to be eliminated from the blood stream. Each subsequent drink if taken within this time will raise the blood alcohol level even further. If a person drinks four units, that is two pints of ordinary lager (or the equivalent amount of alcohol) this is likely to remain in the blood stream for approximately four hours. Care needs to be taken with special lagers since some of these are twice as strong as weaker brews.

Alcohol effects women a little differently from men. Females feel the effects of lower doses of alcohol than men and they also develop problems at approximately a half to two thirds of the alcohol consumption of their male counterparts. It is also clear that women develop problems earlier in their drinking careers than men and although many of the resulting problems are similar the importance put on the problems differs between the genders.

Longer term problems can be divided into three groups:

- Physical;
- Social;
- Legal.

Physical problems include harm such as damage to all the systems in the body, for example:

- *Cardiovascular system* – cardiac damage;
- *Gastrointestinal system* – gastritis, ulcers, pancreatitis, hepatic cirrhosis;
- *Central nervous system* – neuritis, 'black-outs', cerebral atrophy;
- *Genitourinary system* – impotence, subfertility, infertility and in high doses, possibly fetal harm.

An important physical problem is alcohol dependence. For most people this only develops after years of regular heavy drinking. Even so people may become 'psychologically dependent' upon using alcohol as a prop after very short periods. Social problems include harm due to intoxication such as drunken driving and aggressive unpredictable behaviour problems in the home such as spouse battering and child abuse or neglect. More recently the long established link between drinking and unsafe sexual practices has become a greater cause for concern due to the advent of HIV infection. Evidence suggests that people who have been drinking or using other drugs are less likely to use barrier protection during intercourse and more likely to indulge in 'higher risk' sexual practices (Stall *et al* 1986; Robertson and Plant 1988).

Legal problems include a wide range of crimes of 'disinhibition'. These range from public drunkenness to violence, homicide and rape, drinking and driving. Alcohol consumption is associated with many crimes. Even so the connection between drinking and crime is complex and it is often unclear to what extent alcohol contributes to specific criminal acts. It should be noted that being over the legal blood alcohol limit occurs not only when the pubs close in the evening. Someone who has consumed a large quantity of alcohol the previous evening may still be 'over the limit' for driving when he or she sets off for work the next morning.

■ The effects of tobacco

There are many differences between alcohol and tobacco consumption. The most relevant difference here is that small amounts of alcohol have not been shown to be harmful even over long periods of time. However consumption of even small amounts of tobacco increases both morbidity and mortality.

□ Problems with tobacco

Tobacco related harm is mainly physical, for example increased incidence of cancer. In the UK, as in a number of other European countries and in some states in the USA, there is a trend for lung cancer to overtake breast cancer as the leading cause of such deaths amongst women. It was recently pointed out that, 'Scottish women who smoke more than English women and men are in the unenviable position of leading the women's world lung cancer league. American women come a close second' (Jacobson 1988).

Women who smoke are more likely to develop cancers of the upper respiratory and digestive tracts than non-smokers. Furthermore, 'We can now add cervical cancer to the list of tobacco-caused diseases' (Austen 1983).

Heart disease is also more common among women who smoke 20

cigarettes a day or more than amongst other women. The former are twice as likely to die of a heart attack than non-smokers (Jacobson 1988).

■ Alcohol and tobacco

Alcohol is one of the most commonly used psychoactive drugs in the world. For the majority of people who drink in moderation there are no long term or serious ill effects. Tobacco is also a widely used drug. Even so, smoking, even in moderation, is known to cause physical damage not only to the smoker but to her or his associates who inhale tobacco smoke whether they wish to or not.

In the UK, the level of alcohol consumption in the general population virtually doubled between 1950 and 1979 (Taylor 1981). More recently alcohol consumption has declined slightly. Evidence from surveys carried out at different times in different areas over the UK clarify the picture. In 1972 a Scottish survey was carried out by Dight (1976). This showed that 46 per cent of women were regular (weekly) drinkers. Women of higher socioeconomic status and younger women were more commonly regular drinkers (74 per cent of 'professional' women compared with 38 per cent of those from semi- and unskilled manual backgrounds). This study also emphasised the link between smoking and drinking. The group of women who were most likely to drink every week were those who smoked 25 cigarettes or more each day. The average alcohol consumption for women in this study was 4.8 units (See Fig. 5.1).

Another survey (Wilson 1980) indicated that women (aged 20 years and over) in England and Wales who were drinkers consumed a weekly average of 7 units. Women in Scotland consumed a slightly lower average of 6.2 units. In the same year Harbison and Hare (1980) published findings from a Northern Ireland survey. This showed women who drank, consumed an average of 6.5 units weekly. A review by Hilton (1988) of American drinking habits covered eleven surveys carried out between 1964 and 1984.

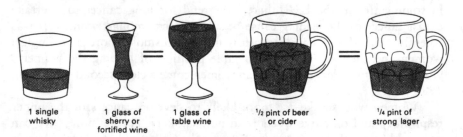

| 1 single whisky | 1 glass of sherry or fortified wine | 1 glass of table wine | ½ pint of beer or cider | ¼ pint of strong lager |

Figure 5.1 What is a unit of alcohol?

By 1984 men were three times more likely to report frequent and heavy drinking or drunkenness than their female counterparts. It is important to stress the fact that these figures relate to drinkers only, because the number of abstainers in a community can make a great difference to the average alcohol consumption of the population. Hilton's review also showed there had been very little change in the percentage of American women classed as abstainers. The latter ranged from 39 per cent to 47 per cent in the studies reviewed. Ahlstrom's (1987) review of women's drinking habits in Finland showed a marked decrease in abstinence between 1968 and 1976. This contrasted with the trend between 1976 and 1984 when abstinence rates rose, but still remained lower than in 1968.

In all areas of the UK women are more likely to be abstainers or infrequent drinkers than are males. In 1985 a study of approximately 2000 women in England and Wales showed 8 per cent were abstainers (Breeze 1985). Interestingly this study also showed the group most likely to be heavy drinkers were young, unmarried, career-oriented women. If this particular trend continues then the next few years may show an increased number of relatively heavy drinkers presenting for antenatal care. Bearing in mind that people who drink heavily often also smoke heavily it is time to heighten the awareness of professional groups such as midwives to the risks of these behaviours.

Recent trends in tobacco consumption in the UK are more encouraging from the perspective of health. It became 'fashionable' for women to smoke after World War I and this trend continued well into the 1950s. By this time more than 40 per cent of women in the UK smoked cigarettes. Since 1972, however, there has been a steady decline in tobacco use. A survey published in 1985 by the Office of Population Censuses and Surveys showed that, by 1984, 32 per cent of women were cigarette smokers compared to 36 per cent of men. Several British surveys have indicated that teenage girls are more likely to smoke than are teenage boys. Even so fewer than 40 per cent do so. However Jarvis (1984) re-examined data from the General Household Survey (OPCS 1985) and also data from similar surveys in the USA, he states that the difference may be more to do with the fact that men stop smoking cigarettes *but* may change to cigar or pipe smoking. Women on the other hand simply stop. Jarvis concludes '... data from Great Britain supported by the experience in the United States, strongly suggests that the sex difference in smoking cessation in the general population is more apparent than real. ... When allowance is made for the differential impact of secondary cigar smoking in men, there is no sex difference in smoking cessation below the age of 50' (page 387).

The message, at least for women, is positive: many can and do give up smoking and are doing so. Smokers of both genders are becoming more and more of a minority. This has already led to a decline in a number of tobacco-related diseases amongst some sub-groups of the population.

■ Alcohol consumption during pregnancy

Discussion of the potential harm of drinking during pregnancy can be traced to ancient times and may be found in historical documents from different countries and different religions (Plant 1987). For centuries it was believed that whatever the pregnant woman saw would affect her baby for good or ill. The Romans and Greeks encouraged their pregnant women to look at beautiful paintings and sculptures. Similarly, when John Merrick (better known as the 'Elephant Man') grew up he was firmly convinced that the reason for his deformities was because his mother had been frightened by a rampaging circus elephant when she had been pregnant. As time progressed people began to discriminate between different types of alcohol. In the UK, by the 18th Century, people were strongly in favour of 'the beneficial effects of beer' but very much against gin and other 'spirituous liquors'. In 1781 a well known professor of midwifery in Dublin highlighted two contradictions which so often beset midwifery when he stated that 'uterine haemorrhage leading to miscarriage or abortion could result from the abuse of stimulants, vinous and other strong liquors' but went on to recommend alcohol as a pain killer in labour (Warner & Rosett 1975). It was still believed at this time, and for a great many years, that the placenta formed a highly effective 'barrier' against any substance likely to harm the fetus. It took on an almost magical quality of being able to differentiate between what was good for the fetus and what was not. It is only in recent years that we have learnt that what passes through the placenta has more to do with molecular weight than with magic.

There have been a number of clear descriptions of babies apparently harmed by their mothers' drinking. A select committee of the House of Commons reported in 1834 'Infants born to alcoholic mothers have a starved, shrivelled and imperfect look' (Warner & Rosett 1975). In fact the certainty with which this pronouncement was made shows how even in days gone by governments could 'get it wrong'. Alcohol was and is only one of many drugs used in the UK. Children born to opium using mothers (also a legal drug at that time) had a strikingly similar description 'the poor, wizened, ill-nourished infants are really pitiable to behold' (Berridge & Edwards, 1981).

At the turn of the century in America, the UK and the rest of Europe other priorities took precedence. The Temperance Movement, from which sprang the Women's Movement both in the US and the UK, was in full swing followed by World War I, Prohibition in the US, and then World War II. It was not till the late 1960s when Lemoine and his colleagues in France published a paper in a French language journal that the debate began again (Lemoine et al 1968). A few years later a paper in The Lancet named the group of clinical features the 'fetal alcohol syndrome' (Jones & Smith 1973).

It is important to state that this syndrome was originally described on the basis of evidence from a group of only eight children, whose mothers were alcohol abusers and also relatively poor with all the concommitant problems which may arise from that state. The fact that these women were atypical was stressed by Jones and Smith, but has subsequently been ignored.

The features of the fetal alcohol syndrome (FAS) are noted below:

PERCENT OCCURRENCE OF ABNORMALITIES

		0 25 50 75 100 %
PERFORMANCE	PRENATAL GROWTH DEFICIENCY	100
	POSTNATAL GROWTH DEFICIENCY	100
	DEVELOPMENTAL DELAY	100
CRANIOFACIES	MICROCEPHALY	91
	SHORT PALPEBRAL FISSURES	100
	EPICANTHAL FOLDS	36
	MAXILLARY HYPOPLASIA	64
	CLEFT PALATE	18
	MICROGNATHIA	27
LIMBS	JOINT ANOMALIES	73
	ALTERED PALMAR CREASE PATTERN	73
OTHER	CARDIAC ANOMALIES	70
	ANOMALOUS EXTERNAL GENITALIA	36
	CAPILLARY HEMANGIOMATA	36
	FINE–MOTOR DYSFUNCTION	80

Source: Jones & Smith (1975)
Figure 5.2 Pattern of malformation in fetal alcohol syndrome

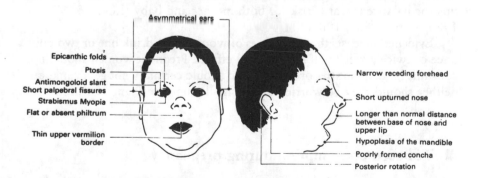

Source: Plant, M.L. (1987)
Figure 5.3 Features of the fetal alcohol syndrome

In an effort to clarify the role of alcohol in pregnancy four large scale studies were set up in the US. The results of these are published elsewhere (Rosett & Weiner 1984). The main findings were surprisingly similar to those reported by Plant (1988a): 'heavy' or problem drinkers had an elevated risk of producing babies with features ranging from low birthweight, difficulty with feeding and sleeping, to fully developed FAS. There appeared to be little evidence, however, that consumption of moderate to low doses of alcohol had adverse effects on the fetus. The major exception to these findings was the work carried out by the team of Streissguth *et al* in 1977. Little (1977) reported a study which showed a link between moderate alcohol consumption and low birthweight. Sadly, in 1981, before these findings were published, the US Surgeon General issued a statement which was to confuse and inflate the issue. This warned of the consumption of alcohol by pregnant women, but it did not specify the fact that it was women who were alcohol abusers or 'alcoholic' who might put themselves and their babies at risk. Instead the statement concluded: 'Each patient should be told about the risks of alcohol consumption during pregnancy and advised not to drink alcoholic beverages and to be aware of the alcoholic content of foods and drugs' (United States Surgeon General 1981).

Debate continues about whether or not pregnant women should give up drinking altogether. Some commentators have suggested that women should abstain even before becoming pregnant (Little *et al* 1982). Alternatively, perhaps drinking during pregnancy is only a problem for those atypical women with alcohol-related problems.

The publication of the four major US studies and numerous others from many countries leads to broadly reassuring conclusions. There seems no doubt that heavy alcohol consumption is risky for pregnant women as indeed it is for anyone. The question of whether alcohol in itself causes fetal harm is still being debated. At the moment many alcohol researchers are inclining towards the theory that it may be the general lifestyle of the problem drinker including factors such as poor nutrition, possible use of tobacco and other drugs combined with stress together with alcohol which tips the balance towards risk for both mother and baby (Rosett & Weiner 1984, Plant 1988a, 1988b).

Evidence suggests that the babies of women who drink one or two units once or twice a week will not suffer ill-effects. Pregnant women should not consume large quantities of alcohol, and should certainly not get drunk, but neither should they be worried about small amounts (Plant 1987).

■ Tobacco consumption during pregnancy

The case against tobacco is clear. Even for women taking steps to avoid pregnancy, by using oral contraceptives for example, the risks are greater for smokers than for non-smokers. For example, as one researcher claims, 'Oral contraceptive use alone does not constitute a significant risk factor for coronary heart disease, but combined with smoking the relative risk is about 12 to 1' (Gritz 1980).

Problems of subfertility, infertility and problems during pregnancy are also well established. In 1980 the US Surgeon General published a report entitled, *The Health Consequences of Smoking in Women*. This report states that, 'the risk of spontaneous abortion, fetal death and neonatal death increases directly with increasing levels of maternal smoking' (US Department of Health and Human Services 1980). The report goes on to describe the smokers' increased risks during pregnancy (for example, threatened abortion), during labour (for example, premature rupture of the membranes, abruptio placentae, placenta praevia) and during breastfeeding (for example, where smoking may affect the supply of breast milk). However the latter effect has not yet been clarified. Stimmel (1982) noted that:

> Smoking during pregnancy has been strongly associated with decreases in fetal birth weight and placenta lesions, as well as an excessive rate of spontaneous abortion and perinatal death (Lowe, C R 1959; Kline, J, *et al* 1977; Naeye, R L 1978). Perinatal mortality has been reported to be 27% higher in smokers as a group than in non-smokers, with adverse placental conditions such as placenta previa and abruptio placentae, to be increased by 28% to 50% in smokers as compared to non-smokers (Fielding, J E 1978).

A large scale study of 51490 births was carried out by Meyer and Tonascia (1977). A summary of the findings by Gritz (1980) stated that:

> Smoking was significantly related to an increase of bleeding during pregnancy, abruptio placentae, placenta praevia and premature and prolonged rupture of the membranes. ... Smokers incurred a threefold greater risk of premature rupture of the membranes for births occurring before 34 weeks gestation, and this risk remained higher through term.

Babies born to smoking mothers are more likely to be 'small-for-dates'. Gritz (1980) points out that 'Because low birthweight is associated with increased infant mortality, the infants of cigarette smokers, who are lighter than those of non-smokers at a given gestational age, have a higher mortality risk. The association between smoking and infant mortality holds when adjustment is made for other risk factors influencing mortality rates.' So regardless of what else the smoking mother ingests, it is the tobacco which seems to cause the harm.

■ Health education

Although pregnancy is an ideal time to inform and encourage women to avoid risky behaviour, there is some evidence from other populations which suggests that simply giving information is not enough (Plant 1987).

Most health education literature is aimed at literate white people in socioeconomic groups 2 and 3. Unfortunately, it is still uncommon to see health education couched in a form which takes into account people's lifestyle, background, religious beliefs and differing levels of education. Anyone who has difficulty with reading will find most health education leaflets to be of little or no value. In fact many health-threatening behaviours (such as smoking) are particularly likely to be seen in people from lower socioeconomic backgrounds. The combination of low income or unemployment and poor housing is associated with many problems in this disadvantaged group.

Another important issue rarely addressed by health professionals was highlighted in the studies carried out by Graham in the UK. Her series of studies started with women's experiences during pregnancy and continued through early motherhood and pre-school years. She states, 'these surveys suggest, first, that risk-taking behaviour cannot be explained in terms of women's ignorance and irresponsibility, and second, that the majority of women have neither the resources nor the opportunity to adopt health-promoting lifestyles for themselves or their families' (Graham 1988). The deficiencies of health education related to psychoactive drugs have been emphasized by Plant (1987): 'Health education is potentially important. Even so, in relation to alcohol, tobacco and prescribed drugs, it must be regarded as purely experimental and should be approached cautiously and with due regard to the evidence that it may be ineffective or harmful.'

Health education is not a panacea for all ills. Unhealthy behaviours are caused by a profusion of factors some of which may be difficult, even impossible, to counter.

It must also be stressed that pregnant women are particularly vulnerable and therefore care should be taken to provide accurate information without exaggerating the health risks of specific behaviours. This is certainly the case with alcohol. In the words of Griffith Edwards (1983) one of the UK's leading drug and alcohol researchers: 'Alcohol problems notoriously attract absolutism, and covert moral stances easily become confused with medical advice. Threats to the unborn child excite particular anxiety.'

■ Recommendations for clinical practice in the light of currently available evidence

1. The task of the midwife in this situation is initially to collect clear information about the alcohol and tobacco consumption of the pregnant woman at the first appointment after the positive pregnancy result.

2. Information should be collected in a way which allows the woman to ask and receive information. One of the most accurate ways of collecting information about drinking is to ask the woman what she has had to drink in terms of alcohol over the past seven days, starting the day prior to the appointment and working backwards. This usually gives a reasonably accurate picture of the previous week's consumption. Using the rule of thumb 'One or two units once or twice a week' it can be assessed whether recommendations for reduction in consumption would be necessary. If so helpful hints are in order (see Fig. 5.4). However the midwife should be aware that the pregnant woman is on the 'midwife's territory', not her own, and her anxiety level will be high. It is therefore important not only to discuss some possible ways of helping reduce consumption but also to follow this up with written information (Robertson & Heather 1985) and to make a note in the case-notes to ask for any problems at subsequent visits.

---

1. Don't drink daily, give yourself five or six days in the week drink free
2. Make every second drink alcohol-free or low alcohol
3. Sip your drink, don't gulp
4. Always lay your glass down between sips
5. Above all don't get into 'tangles' or arguments with people who press drinks on you. Make it clear from the outset that neither you nor your baby want to drink any more. This, with a firm 'Thank you', will usually do the trick!

Figure 5.4 Helpful hints for reducing alcohol consumption

3. The majority of people who smoke and drink will say that it is more difficult to give up tobacco than alcohol. However there are some 'helpful hints' for smokers too. For instance it is going to be easier for the pregnant women to stop smoking if her partner also stops. This not only gives mutual support but helps remove the temptation. One of the most successful methods of stopping smoking is to set a date and stick to it. Ideally this date should occur during a period when the triggers which lead to smoking (for example stress) are at their lowest. To aid this decision, the woman should then identify the times of day, situations and company which are most likely to encourage her to smoke – for example breakfast, morning tea break, etc. This identification could usefully be worked out with the midwife at the clinic.

4. The woman should be encouraged to compliment or reward herself initially each day she remains a non-smoker. This is a time when helpful friends can give encouragement. Last but not least she should be aware of now looking for no-smoking areas in public places; that way someone else's smoke will not be so tempting.

5. Clearly there is not time for the midwife in the clinic to go over all the issues on changing these habits. Even so, acknowledgement of the possible difficulties and some guidelines such as sitting down and consciously identifying 'high risk' times may be one of the most useful ways in which to help the woman to focus her mind. When she is desperate for a cigarette, she may find it easier to picture her baby happy and healthy as the reward for not having one.

6. Any goal setting such as cutting alcohol consumption to one or two units once or twice a week or stopping smoking must be done by the woman after negotiation between the woman and the midwife. This ensures that the goals set are attainable and reduces the risk of failure. With smoking cessation in particular the woman may need a great deal of support.

7. The fact that the woman is a smoker will obviously be recorded in the notes. If she decides to stop smoking, she should be praised and acknowledgement of her success should be given at each visit. However it must be stressed that if she fails criticism won't help. Even a reduction in tobacco consumption is beneficial for her baby. It must also be noted that pregnant women with other young children at home will have an extremely difficult task trying to stop smoking. As Graham (1988) writes, 'being responsible [*viz* giving up smoking] involved not simply meeting the needs of the unborn baby, but reconciling these needs with those of other members of the family. Reconciling needs demanded the constant presence and attention of the mother – and smoking offered a way of temporarily escaping without leaving the room.' Just as the unborn child should not be romanticised the difficulties involved in giving up smoking should not be minimised. If they are, the expectant mother may feel a failure and when she experiences difficulties she will not be able to share these problems. If this happens the opportunity of continued support from the midwife may be lost.

■ Practice check

The questions which the midwife asks herself on this topic are not as simple as in other areas. They are questions such as:

- 'How do I feel about someone who drinks too much woman?'

- 'Do I treat people with these types of problems with care?'

- 'How do I feel if people do not seem willing or able advice?'

- 'Do I give up and just ignore them or can I remain positive even if small steps are taken to change behaviour?'

Most difficult of all given the number of nurses and midwives who smoke:

- 'How do I *comfortably* explain to someone that smoking is unsafe not only for her baby but also for herself when I've just come from my coffee break?'

Remember the smell of smoke lingers on clothes and hands. People are more likely to copy what you *do* than what you say.

Being human and acknowledging difficulties often makes it much easier for the pregnant woman to view you as an approachable support person. It is only honest to acknowledge that most of us have difficulty in giving up immediate or short-term pleasures for long-term benefits.

☐ **Acknowledgements**

Acknowledgements are made to the Scottish Health Education Group and Drs Jones and Smith of the School of Medicine, Seattle.

■ References

Ahlstrom S 1987 Women's use of alcohol. In Simpura J (ed) Finnish drinking habits. Finnish Foundation for Alcohol Studies, Helsinki

Austen D F 1983 Smoking and cervical cancer. Journal of the American Medical Association 250 (4): 515–17

Berridge V, Edwards G 1981 Opium and the people: 104. Allen Lane, London

Breeze E 1985 Women and drinking. HMSO, London

Dadak C, Leithner C, Sinzinger H, Silberbauer K 1981 Diminished prostacyclin formation in umbilical arteries of babies born to women who smoke. Lancet i: 94

Dight S 1976 Scottish drinking habits. HMSO, London

Edwards G 1983 Alcohol and advice to pregnant women. British Medical Journal 286: 247–48

An... Smoking and pregnancy. New England J...
298: 337–39

F.., Carpenter C W 1973 Induction in mid trimester ...
intra-uterine alcohol. Obstetrics and Gynaecology 41(5).

...aham H 1998 Health ... In McPherson A (ed) Wome...
general practice ...–51. Oxford University Press, Oxford

Glitz E R 1984 Problems related to the use of tobacco by wome...
(ed) Alcohol and drug problems in women: Research advanc...
and drug problems Vol 5: 487–513. Plenum Press, New York.

Harbison J, Haran T 1980 Drinking in Northern Ireland. Social Research
Public Policy Unit, Belfast

Hilton M E 1998 Trends in US drinking patterns. further evidence from
20 years. British Journal of Addiction 83: 269–79

Jacobson B 1988 Beating the ladykillers. Women and smoking. Gollancz.

Jarvis M 1984 Cinder and smoking. do women really find it harder to giv...
British Journal of Addiction 79: 383, 87

Jones K L, Smith D W 1973 Recognition of the fetal alcohol syndrome in early
infancy. Lancet ii: 999, 1001

Jones K L, Smith D W 1975 The fetal alcohol syndrome. Teratology 12: 1–10

Kline J, Stein Z A, Susser M 1977 Smoking. a risk factor for spontaneous
abortions. New England Journal of Medicine 297: 793–96

Lole A S 1992 Fetal alcohol syndrome: other effects of alcohol on pregnancy.
New York State Journal of Medicine July: 1125–37

Lemoine P, Harousseau H, Borteyru J P, Menuet J C 1968 Enfants de parents
alcooliques: anomalies observées à propos 127 cas. Ouest Medicale
25: 476–82

Little R E 1977 Moderate alcohol use during pregnancy and decreased infant
birthweight. American Journal of Public Health 67: 1154–56

Little R E, Graham J M, Samson H H 1982 Fetal alcohol effects in humans and
animals, In Stimmel B (ed) The effects of maternal alcohol and drug abuse on
the newborn. The Haworth Press, New York

Lowe C R 1959 Effects of mothers' smoking habits on birthweight of their
children. British Medical Journal 2: 673–76

Marsh A, Dobbs J, White A 1986 Adolescent drinking. HMSO, London

Manning F A, Feyerabend C 1976 Cigarette smoking and foetal breathing
movements. British Journal of Obstetrics and Gynaecology 83: 262–70

Meyer M B, Tonascia J A 1977 Maternal smoking, pregnancy complications and
perinatal mortality. American Journal of Obstetrics and Gynecology
128: 494–505

Naeye R L 1978 Effects of maternal cigarette smoking on the fetus and the
placenta. British Journal of Obstetrics and Gynaecology 85: 732–35

Office of Population Censuses and Surveys 1985 Drinking and attitudes to
licensing in Scotland. HMSO, London

Plant M A 1987 Drugs in perspective. Hodder and Stoughton, London

Plant M L 1987 Women drinking and pregnancy. Tavistock Publications, London

Plant M L 1988a Drinking and pregnancy: a review. International Clinical
Nutrition Review 8 (1): 19–21

Plant M L 1988b Drink problems. In McPherson A (ed) Women's problems in
general practice: 402–19. Oxford University Press, Oxford

Fielding J E 1978 Smoking and pregnancy. New England Journal of
    Medicine   298: 337–39
Gomel V, Carpenter C W 1973 Induction of mid-trimester abortion with
    intra-uterine alcohol. Obstetrics and Gynaecology   41(3): 455–58
Graham H 1988 Health education. In McPherson A (ed) Women's problems in
    general practice: 438–51. Oxford University Press, Oxford
Gritz E R 1980 Problems related to the use of tobacco by women. In Kalant O J
    (ed) Alcohol and drug problems in women: Research advances in alcohol
    and drug problems Vol 5: 487–543. Plenum Press, New York, London
Harbison J, Hare T 1980 Drinking in Northern Ireland. Social Research Division
    Public Policy Unit, Belfast
Hilton M E 1988 Trends in US drinking patterns: further evidence from the past
    20 years. British Journal of Addiction   83: 269–78
Jacobson B 1988 Beating the ladykillers: women and smoking. Gollancz, London
Jarvis M 1984 Gender and smoking: do women really find it harder to give up?
    British Journal of Addiction   79: 383–87
Jones K L, Smith D W 1973 Recognition of the fetal alcohol syndrome in early
    infancy. Lancet   ii: 999–1001
Jones K L, Smith D W 1975 The fetal alcohol syndrome. Teratology   12: 1–10
Kline J, Stein Z A, Susser M 1977 Smoking: a risk factor for spontaneous
    abortions. New England Journal of Medicine   297: 793–96
Lele A S 1982 Fetal alcohol syndrome: other effects of alcohol on pregnancy.
    New York State Journal of Medicine   July: 1225–27
Lemoine P, Harronsseau H, Borteyru J P, Menuet J C 1968 Enfants de parents
    alcooliques: anomalies observées à propos 127 cas. Quest Medicale
    25: 476–82
Little R E 1977 Moderate alcohol use during pregnancy and decreased infant
    birthweight. American Journal of Public Health   67: 1154–56
Little R E, Graham J M, Samson H H 1982 Fetal alcohol effects in humans and
    animals, In Stimmel B (ed) The effects of maternal alcohol and drug abuse on
    the newborn. The Haworth Press, New York
Lowe C R 1959 Effects of mothers' smoking habits on birthweight of their
    children. British Medical Journal   2: 673–76
Marsh A, Dobbs J, White A 1986 Adolescent drinking. HMSO, London
Manning F A, Feyerabend C 1976 Cigarette smoking and foetal breathing
    movements. British Journal of Obstetrics and Gynaecology   83: 262–70
Meyer M B, Tonascia J A 1977 Maternal smoking, pregnancy complications and
    perinatal mortality. American Journal of Obstetrics and Gynecology
    128: 494–505
Naeye R L 1978 Effects of maternal cigarette smoking on the fetus and the
    placenta. British Journal of Obstetrics and Gynaecology   85: 732–35
Office of Population Censuses and Surveys 1985 Drinking and attitudes to
    licensing in Scotland. HMSO, London
Plant M A 1987 Drugs in perspective. Hodder and Stoughton, London
Plant M L 1987 Women drinking and pregnancy. Tavistock Publications, London
Plant M L 1988a Drinking and pregnancy: a review. International Clinical
    Nutrition Review   8 (1): 19–21
Plant M L 1988b Drink problems. In McPherson A (ed) Women's problems in
    general practice: 402–19. Oxford University Press, Oxford

- 'How do I feel about someone who drinks too much; particularly a woman?'

- 'Do I treat people with these types of problems with less respect or care?'

- 'How do I feel if people do not seem willing or able to act on my advice?'

- 'Do I give up and just ignore them or can I remain positive even if small steps are taken to change behaviour?'

Most difficult of all given the number of nurses and midwives who smoke:

- 'How do I *comfortably* explain to someone that smoking is unsafe not only for her baby but also for herself when I've just come from my coffee break?'

Remember the smell of smoke lingers on clothes and hands. People are more likely to copy what you *do* than what you say.

Being human and acknowledging difficulties often makes it much easier for the pregnant woman to view you as an approachable support person. It is only honest to acknowledge that most of us have difficulty in giving up immediate or short-term pleasures for long-term benefits.

□ Acknowledgements

Acknowledgements are made to the Scottish Health Education Group and Drs Jones and Smith of the School of Medicine, Seattle.

■ References

Ahlstrom S 1987 Women's use of alcohol. In Simpura J (ed) Finnish drinking habits. Finnish Foundation for Alcohol Studies, Helsinki

Austen D F 1983 Smoking and cervical cancer. Journal of the American Medical Association 250 (4): 515–17

Berridge V, Edwards G 1981 Opium and the people: 104. Allen Lane, London

Breeze E 1985 Women and drinking. HMSO, London

Dadak C, Leithner C, Sinzinger H, Silberbauer K 1981 Diminished prostacyclin formation in umbilical arteries of babies born to women who smoke. Lancet i: 94

Dight S 1976 Scottish drinking habits. HMSO, London

Edwards G 1983 Alcohol and advice to pregnant women. British Medical Journal 286: 247–48

Robertson I, Heather N 1985 So you want to cut down your drinking? Scottish Health Education Group, Edinburgh

Robertson J A, Plant M L 1988 Alcohol, sex and risks of HIV infection. Drug and Alcohol Dependence 22: 75–8

Rosett H L, Weiner L 1984 Alcohol and the fetus. Oxford University Press, New York

Rush D, Cassano P 1983 Relationship of cigarette smoking and social class to birthweight and perinatal mortality. Journal of Epidemiology and Community Health 37: 249–55

Stall R, McKusick L, Wiley J *et al* 1986 Alcohol and drug use during sexual activity and compliance with safe sex guidelines for AIDS. Health Education Quarterly 13: 359–71

Stimmel B (ed) 1982 The effects of maternal alcohol and drug abuse in the newborn. Haworth Press, New York

Taylor D 1981 Alcohol: reducing the harm. Office of Health Economics, London

United States Department of Health and Human Services 1980 The health consequences of smoking for women. Rockville MD

United States Surgeon General 1981 Advisory on alcohol and pregnancy. Food and Drug Administration Bulletin 1 (2): 9–10

Van Vunakis H, Langone J J, Milunsky A 1974 Nicotine and cotinine in the amniotic fluid of smokers in the second trimester of pregnancy. American Journal of Obstetrics and Gynecology 120: 64–6

Warner R H, Rosett H L 1975 The effects of drinking on offspring. Journal of Studies on Alcohol 36 (11): 1395–420

Wilson P 1980 Drinking in England and Wales. HMSO, London

■ Suggested further reading

Kalant O J (ed) 1980 Alcohol and drug problems in women. Plenum Press, New York, London

Plant M L 1987 Women, drinking and pregnancy. Tavistock Publications, London

Rosett H L, Weiner L, 1984 Alcohol and the fetus. Oxford University Press, New York

Wilsnack S C, Beckman L J 1984 Alcohol problems in women. Guildford Press, New York

Chapter 6

Antenatal education

Tricia Murphy-Black

Good teaching is easy to recognise but not always easy to achieve. Antenatal education is a particular challenge as the midwife has little choice over the attenders, the group will be varied in their ages and their knowledge, connected only by the one event they have in common. Teaching pregnant women consists of approaching a sensitive subject in which they are deeply involved and about which they may have strong feelings. The most effective teaching will be that which focuses on the interests of those who attend, so they are given the opportunity to learn what they want to learn.

Although there has been antenatal education for many years, the challenge is greater in the 1980s and 1990s. Parents today are a sophisticated group who have been watching professional presentations on television all their lives, who are accustomed to being enticed by advertisements, and whose education has involved a variety of methods and approaches. As a result those parents who are not interested in the classes will vote with their feet and leave. If it is generally known that the classes do not meet the needs of parents, they will not even start attending.

It has been assumed for some years that a midwife, because she is a midwife, has the ability to teach (Myles 1975) but this has been challenged more recently (Sayle 1979). Although much of midwifery does involve teaching, the main skills are those of one-to-one teaching; teaching a group demands different skills which can and should be learned.

■ **It is assumed that you are already aware of the following:**

● How to teach (you should have been given the basic skills during your training);

● Basic knowledge of communication skills and how to use them;

> - Clients did not want to go
> - Clients did not know about classes
> - Clients thought classes not worthwhile
> - Clients thought exercises might harm baby
> - Clients felt confident without attending
> - Too costly
> - Poor timing in the day
> - Poor transport or location difficult
> - Clients attended in previous pregnancy
> - No provision for children

Sources: RCM 1966; Gillett 1976; Perkins 1978b; Homans 1980; Boyd & Sellars 1982; McCabe *et al* 1984; McIntosh 1988

Figure 6.1 Factors attributed to poor attendance at antenatal classes

- Which skills are required in the management of group dynamics;

- Different approaches to health promotion – of which you will need to select an appropriate one. It may be useful to inform mothers of those behaviours which are harmful; those which benefit and those which are just individual choice, so it is clear that the choices are for the individual woman to make;

- That antenatal education has to meet the needs of the parents if it is to be of any value.

■ Antenatal education – critical appraisal of the literature

Antenatal education in the UK developed from two separate traditions. The first aimed to educate parents about hygiene and general baby care as part of the strategy to reduce the high perinatal and infant mortality at the beginning of the 20th century (Williams & Booth 1974). The second tradition focused on methods to alleviate pain in labour, with the use of various methods such as physical relaxation, the natural childbirth movement of Dick-Read, hypnosis, psychoprophylaxis and, in the later part of this century, acupuncture (Kitzinger 1972; Williams & Booth 1974; Williamson 1975; Heardman 1982; Skelton 1984). With the recognition of the importance of antenatal care during World War II, it was possible to establish mothercraft classes throughout the country when the NHS was introduced in 1948. Provision has varied through the years but, in the late 1980s, classes are available in most maternity units with many community midwives and health visitors providing classes in the local clinics.

☐ **Benefits of antenatal education**

Antenatal education has been the focus of research for many years. Investigations into the effectiveness of physical preparation for childbirth have produced conflicting results. Benefits, such as a reduction in the use of analgesic drugs (Roberts *et al* 1953) and increased confidence in labour (Rathbone 1973) have been demonstrated. Breathing and relaxation were the most effective form of pain relief in a group of mothers who did not have epidural analgesia (Taylor 1985). Assessment with the McGill Pain Questionnaire (Niven 1984) showed that attendance at classes was associated with lower pain levels on part of the assessment. Others have reported, however, that antenatal education has little influence on the course or the outcome of labour (Rodway 1947; Burnett 1956; Mandelstram 1971) nor could exercises alone result in painless childbirth (McKenna 1976).

Other benefits of class attendance have been more difficult to measure. The confidence reported by Rathbone (1973) did not always last throughout labour and only a small reduction of anxiety and increased knowledge was found by Hibbard *et al* (1979). Ball (1981) identified a 'distressed' group of mothers, reporting that 62.2 per cent of them had attended classes compared with 37.2 per cent of those mothers who were in the 'high satisfaction' group. It might be argued that those who were more likely to be distressed would choose to attend classes, and those who would be satisfied with their childbirth experience might choose not to attend. A difference in the mothers may also explain Orr's (1980) demonstration of a significant relationship between those not attending classes and the subsequent under utilisation of well baby clinics. Husband (1983) showed that clients' educational attainment at the time of booking is a better predictor of attendance at classes than social class.

With the improved standards of living today it could be argued that there is no longer a need to teach about hygiene. Yet the classes, which have come from this tradition, also include the teaching of the skills of baby care, which is appreciated by those women who have not had an opportunity to learn such skills (Taylor 1985). Various researchers have shown that there is much mothers do not know about pregnancy and childcare (RCM 1966; Watson & Morrison 1979; Boyd & Sellars 1982; Morgan 1984; Griffiths & Jenner 1985). Such a need may have been identified but does not appear to have been met as there are a number of studies which show that the mothers learnt little (RCM 1966; Adams 1982), that the information wanted was not covered (Chamberlain 1975; Perkins 1978a), that the preparation covered was not realistic (Draper *et al* 1982), or that the focus was on childbirth and not parenthood (Taylor 1985). Other reports suggest that mothers do find classes to be helpful and to increase their understanding of events (Gillett 1976; Boyd & Sellars 1982; Husband 1983). This may seem encouraging but the research design can be criticised as the Boyd and

Sellars survey was of a self-selected group and Gillett's questions were framed to invite a positive response.

☐ **Attendance at classes**

Attendance at classes has never been high; only about half of all expectant parents go to classes (Burnett 1956; RCM 1966; Laughran 1973; Craig 1981; Amos *et al* 1988). There are more mothers attending classes from the higher social classes (Newson & Newson 1965; O'Brien & Smith 1981; McIntosh 1988) as well as fathers (Taylor 1985). Boswell (1979) in a retrospective study demonstrated no social class difference but reported that those least likely to attend were the younger, single mothers living a distance from the hospital. A national study with a large representative sample had 41 per cent who attended classes (Jacoby 1988). This study confirmed the opinion of many antenatal teachers about the characteristics of attenders; the majority are expecting their first baby, are married, white-caucasian, are owner/occupiers and of the non-manual social class.

The audience has to be attracted, so classes should be advertised more widely (RCM 1966; Perkins 1978a, 1978b). Attempts have been made with posters (Rees 1982), using local press and different languages where appropriate (Greenwood 1983), or information about all the classes within the hospital catchment area and individual written invitations being given out (RCM 1966; Perkins 1978c). Those who will not attend should be taught at clinics (Thomson 1980) with one suggestion to use 'bingo' or 'one armed bandits' to make the education more attractive (Hibbard *et al* 1979).

Despite the small proportion of mothers attending classes, not all were able to complete the course, whether hospital or community based (Breese 1976, Perkins 1978d). Recommendations have been made for classes to be held more frequently towards the end of pregnancy, for mothers to be booked in earlier with some classes held at the beginning of pregnancy, for courses near each other to have staggered starting dates, for classes to be continued for hospital in-patients or planned not to coincide with clinic appointments (RCM 1966; Perkins 1978c; Rees 1982; Taylor 1985). Apart from these suggestions during pregnancy others focused on the postnatal period recommending that some topics, such as family planning, might be more appropriate after the birth of the baby (Perkins 1980a).

☐ **Involving partners**

Antenatal education is now frequently referred to as 'parentcraft'. Both women and their husbands are often keen to participate (Brant 1978) and it is advocated by professionals (Ritchie 1970; Adams 1982). Although prospective fathers might like to attend all classes, often they are only offered one or two classes or a special fathers' evening session (McCabe *et al* 1984; Taylor 1985). This seems to go against the fact they are welcome in the labour ward (Perkins 1980b) and there is some evidence that class attenders are more likely to accompany their partners than non-attenders (Gillett 1976). In 1966, the RCM survey reported that only 10 per cent of fathers were invited to classes but more recent research (Boyd & Sellars 1982) showed an improved figure of 60 per cent. A nationally representative sample in Great Britain showed that more than twice as many partners attending antenatal classes were from the higher (rather than the lower) socioeconomic groups (Farleys 1988).

☐ Prenatal education in North America

Although the system of maternity care in the USA is different from that in the UK, some of the difficulties seen in the UK are also found in America. One report of a hospital in New Jersey (Whitley 1979) describes the 'conventional prenatal class' which is similar to the British parentcraft classes except that relaxation and exercises are only offered as a single optional session. The prepared childbirth classes (PCC) appear to correspond to the National Childbirth Trust (NCT) classes in the UK and are seen as an addition to the hospital classes. As with the NCT in the UK, the parents attending the PCC were better educated and had a higher socio-economic status, they were older, more likely to be nulliparae and intending to breastfeed than those attending the prenatal classes. Demand for the classes was high as it was a requirement for husbands if they wanted to be with their wives during labour and delivery (Whitley 1979). Brown (1982) states that one of the reasons for providing prenatal education is the increased public awareness of the importance of health education.

Enkin (1982), reviewing the medical literature from North America, concluded that the most significant impact of childbirth education is not its effect on the individual mothers but the effect that the availability of such education has in producing significant changes in the ambience in which women give birth. He feels that attendance rates between a third and a half of expectant mothers raises group consciousness so that the well informed consumers influence childbirth practices. Educationalists, also arguing for prenatal education, see evaluation in terms of effect on maternal and infant mortality and morbidity rates (Greenberg & Sullivan 1977). Genest (1981) reports that the benefits of preparation for childbirth are the positive feelings of the parents about childbirth.

Some of the American research has focused on the effectiveness of psychoprophylaxis. Neuromuscular release and practice of breathing techniques were associated with less pain during the active phase of labour (Cogan 1978). Worthington *et al* (1982) examined the influence of active pain control techniques on coping strategies. To test the strategies the subjects' hands were immersed in iced water and length of tolerance and self-reported pain were used as measures of effectiveness. Structured breathing was more useful than normal breathing; effleurage was not helpful but a combination of structured breathing and 'attention focal points' (concentration on a distant point) was more effective than normal breathing. The most effective techniques were the combination of structured breathing, 'attention focal points' and coaching. The disadvantage of this study was that the source of pain was the iced water rather than the contractions of labour. In another more realistic study, mothers who were trained for labour did have less medication than the untrained but the length of labour was longer (Zax *et al* 1975). Conversely a significant reduction in the length of labour was demonstrated in groups of 52 prepared mothers compared with a non-prepared group of 16 mothers (Kuczynski, 1984). The reports of pain experienced during labour relate to the mother's confidence in her preparation as well as the support of her husband. Although much of this confidence may stem from learning skill and attitudes, it is suggested that the social and emotional aspects of classes may be more important (Cogan *et al* 1976).

The American studies indicated that aspects of prenatal education are effective in labour. Cogan (1978) and Worthington *et al* (1982) give a detailed account of the training of mothers, which is more explicit than the British reports of muscular relaxation (Rodway, 1947) and relaxation and controlled breathing (Roberts *et al* 1953). Burnett (1956) also adds exercise of the muscles which will be used in labour. None of these British studies reported a reduction in the length of labour as did Kuczynski (1984), indeed Burnett (1956) noted that labour was longer in the exercised mothers. The disadvantages of Kuczynski's retrospective study which gave little detail of the classes which were successful, were overcome to some extent in a subsequent prospective study of 15 matched pairs of mothers who had and had not attended Lamaze classes. This showed a decrease in anxiety in the prepared group of mothers (Kuczynski & Thompson 1985) which the authors conclude results in prepared patients requiring less of the nurses' time in labour and delivery, which in turn reduces hospital stay and costs.

As a measure, satisfaction with prenatal classes in the US does not appear to suffer from the conflicting results found in the British reports. This review of the American literature is limited and may not present the full picture. Willmuth *et al* (1978) demonstrated that mothers who attended a course for preparation for childbirth, found that their internal locus of control was related to satisfaction with the experience of childbirth. The small number of mothers who completed childbirth education classes had significantly more positive attitudes than those who had only attended one class (Zacharias 1981). Without giving any justification for her statements Whitley (1979) claims classes are a source of satisfaction to everyone. Giefer and Nelson (1981) report a study of teaching fathers which they acknowledge has the limitations of not being controlled, but say that the fathers indicated the classes were effective. Seat belts were the focus of a campaign in some childbirth classes and demonstrated increases in use between 9–11 per cent compared with the classes which acted as controls (Chng *et al* 1987) which implies both learning and change in behaviour.

As in the UK the debate about the approach to teaching is a cause for concern. For instance, Roberts (1976) and Carey (1981) feel teaching should be on a one-to-one basis. Alternatively, participation in prenatal classes is reported as a key factor (Bonovich 1981) in the learning process and that it can be incorporated into classes without disrupting the system or taking up more of the nurses' time. Discussion, role-playing, encounter groups and transactional analysis are recommended in classes described as the psychoprophylactic method (Jiminez 1980). Structured training sessions were favoured to unstructured discussions when teaching expectant fathers but were not evaluated (Campbell & Worthington 1982).

☐ The antenatal teacher

Attention has been paid to the teaching of NHS antenatal classes. Criticism of classes has included poor preparation; giving conflicting advice; not being realistic enough about the burdens of, or giving the wrong impression of parenthood (Breese 1976, Perkins 1978b, Homans 1980; Oakley 1981; Rees 1982; Draper *et al* 1982; Taylor 1985). Antenatal teachers themselves have expressed dissatisfaction. The list of complaints has included:

- The classes are too formal and geared to middle class attenders;

- The classes are offered too late in pregnancy;

- Communication between midwives and health visitors is poor;

- Health visitors especially have complained that their involvement in classes is too sporadic (Rees 1982).

Other complaints have been made about the poor class venues, suitability of accommodation, rigidity of management structures which prevent innovation and a failure to attract parents from all social backgrounds (McCabe *et al* 1984).

Perkins (1981) felt that the problems with the parentcraft teaching were due to the style of teaching when the teachers, rather than the parents, made the decisions about content. Limitations included inadequate identification of the needs of the groups, inadequate control of the topics taught, ineffective teaching, poor staff relationships and lack of flexibility. While management may contribute indirectly by prescribing a rigid syllabus (for instance, Craven *et al* 1975), recent evidence suggests there is more flexibility than there used to be (Burrell 1988). Other difficulties facing teachers is the lack of preparation time and an inability to follow one group of mothers through the course, but even if these are overcome, without training in teaching and group work skills, improvement may be beyond their professional capacities. Group teaching requires different skills and some midwives are aware of these needs. Jamieson (1981, 1982, 1986) has been pleading for team teaching, learning by discussion of emotional aspects, assessment, flexibility within antenatal classes and evaluation at the end of a course.

The midwife has been recognised for many years as having a vital role in teaching (CMB 1962; DHSS 1976; CMB 1980; UKCC 1986) despite the lack of preparation for this role (Ashton 1977; Brammer 1977; Sayle 1979; Sweet 1984). The 18 month midwifery training, which started in 1981, has reduced the percentage of those who felt they were inadequately prepared for their teaching role (Robinson *et al* 1983). The provision for training for this type of teaching is varied, but with increased awareness of the importance of post-basic education, it is hoped that the courses and other opportunities for qualified midwives will be grasped enthusiastically. Midwives and health visitors who had chosen to attend a course aimed at improving their teaching and group work skills had higher levels of interaction with the mothers in the post-course classes compared with the pre-course classes (Murphy-Black 1986).

☐ **Interaction**

Focusing on interaction may seem to be shifting the emphasis of antenatal education away from teaching. Yet without an exchange with the parents it is not possible to know what they want to learn or whether they have learnt anything. Much of midwifery is teaching parents, and midwives are becoming increasingly aware of the need to base their care on what the parents want. Such individualised assessment of the mothers in their care could have two benefits for antenatal education. Midwives who are used to and have the skills of assessment will use these skills in the teaching situation, and that inevitably means that interaction has to occur. The ideal situation would be one where each mother's assessment or birth plan is available for the antenatal teacher so that she knows of the previous experience of the mothers, their needs within the classes, and can form a basis for planning the content of both the sessions and the course. It may be that the only way to achieve this is by the mothers holding their own case notes and bringing them to the classes.

■ **Recommendations for practice in the light of currently available evidence:**

Classes which aim to discuss emotional and sensitive subjects such as pregnancy and the transition to parenthood need to be informal. Antenatal teachers who have learnt under a formal, didactic system may not find it easy to change from knowing in advance what information is to be given by the teacher to groups where 'anything' may be raised, and the 'important' topics are not covered. Yet the sessions where the women's dreams are discussed may be more effective teaching than a detailed lecture, complete with diagrams, of the mechanisms of labour.

1. To be able to create such an atmosphere, the teacher should try to make the surroundings as informal as possible.

2. Have comfortable chairs, or large cushions in a circle or semicircle, rather than rows of hard backed chairs. Discussion is much easier if everyone can see each other.

3. Unless it is impossible, don't wear uniform, it is easier to sit crosslegged on the floor in a track suit. This may take away from the formal position of teacher but aid the feeling that the midwife is a group leader.

4. Using first names to introduce the teacher and each member in the class will not mean loss of position in the group — but it does make it easier for all participants to be friendly and more relaxed.

5. Encourage those in the class to contribute their own experience to help others. This might mean spending some time in the first session getting to know their backgrounds and what their experience has been, not just in relation to pregnancy but other aspects of life. This time is not wasted, even though it may not be covering the syllabus, as it will help the group members to provide mutual support, which may be more important to them than information (Winkler 1988).

6. Use gimmicks if they are a help; these may be ice breakers in the form of games, a list of feelings about childbirth, or antenatal diaries which you have encouraged the group to keep (see Murphy-Black & Faulkner 1987, for further details). Try a 'lucky bag' by using a plastic bag or similar which has a variety of items which may be associated with a particular topic. Each mother is asked to pick something without looking and then takes a turn in guessing what the item is or asking questions about it (Jukes 1988).

7. Provide some form of drink (tea or juice) which provides a break and allows the group members to chat among themselves or gives individual women the opportunity to ask the teacher questions they did not want to ask in front of the rest of the group.

8. Whenever possible, include babies in the group, even if not using them for demonstration purposes. Yes, they will cry and make it

difficult to lecture, but mothers and fathers will participate, ask questions and talk more than in the sessions without babies (Murphy-Black 1986).

9. Be as flexible as possible with visual aids. If the only way to obtain a film on a particular topic is to order it six months in advance, then it might be better not to use it; otherwise it may fix the topic as labour, when the group are full of questions about feeding. If there is a supply of short trigger films, either on video or film, this gives the flexibility to choose what the group want when they want.

10. Prepare any films or videos by viewing them in advance and having some points noted down. Prime the group to look out for one or two points, and then ask questions about these points at the end. This is more useful than a general question like 'what did you think of that?' which could inhibit discussion rather than encourage it.

11. Try team teaching – either with another midwife or a health visitor. This will need some preparation together, but can be very useful if one leads a discussion and the other takes notes of the points which have not come up and can fill in at the end. If the group are discussing the advantages of breastfeeding, for instance, the parents may have given a reasonable list but with one or two items missing. The teacher leading the discussion may be so busy encouraging the quiet ones to contribute and trying to discourage an anecdote that isn't relevant, that she hasn't noted the points that have been missed.

12. Use silence to give mothers the opportunity to talk. One of the difficulties is the feeling that the teacher has to keep things flowing. If there is a silence that goes on too long, it is tempting to fill it with chatter. In classes which were observed and analysed, after asking questions 29 per cent of the teachers paused for less than three seconds before going on talking (Murphy-Black, 1986). There are two ways of helping with this situation. Firstly, the teacher could try timing herself and see how long she can keep quiet; 12 seconds seems like a long time when waiting for a reply but really it is very short. There may be something that can be done to prevent feeling the silent gap, such as glancing at notes, putting a pen away, taking something out of a pocket, looking round at everyone, not just those sitting right in front. Any of these tricks will only take a few seconds but they will stop the feeling of embarrassment and give the group members a chance to think about what they want to say. The other technique is to examine the questions used. Are they unanswerable questions? Is there a plan for using questions? For instance, use closed questions to each member at the beginning so that every one has spoken at least once, even if it is only to say when the baby is

due or whether the baby's father will be with her in labour or not.
Then it is possible to move to more open questions such as

 – 'How do you feel about ...'

and if the answer is short either reflect the answer

 – 'You felt ...?'

or make an encouraging noise. If that doesn't help turn it to other
people

 – 'Did anyone else feel ...'

or use the experience of dealing with other groups

 – 'I remember someone who felt that and she ...'

The question which does not work well is

 – 'Are there any questions?'

In the study mentioned above, this question was asked 150 times in
76 classes. As a technique to encourage mothers to ask questions it
only worked on 17 per cent of occasions (Murphy-Black 1986).

13. In these days of financial constraint, some of these recommendations
may not seem possible. There may have to be compromise to make
the best of a difficult situation. So the comfortable chairs may not be
possible but the pillows for relaxation can be used to get away from
the dreaded rows of chairs. It may not be possible to change the
clinic that coincides with some of the classes, but it may be possible
to change the time of the sessions to follow one group through the
full course. Try to negotiate with the local manager for preparation
time; this should be part of the work associated with teaching. If
there is no formal time with the other teacher it might be possible to
prepare by coming early for the session or before a joint clinic or
spending lunch time together.

■ Practice check

All teachers find it difficult to know whether or not their classes have been
any good. This is perhaps more difficult in antenatal education as there is no
test at the end and, indeed, the parents themselves may not know if the
classes were what they wanted until after the baby is born.

Do you evaluate your classes? If not, you might like to consider some of
the following methods:

● *Postnatal reunion* – Having a postnatal reunion for the parents and
their babies serves two purposes. It will give the mothers an

opportunity to get together again and discuss both their experience of labour and looking after their babies so that they feel less isolated. The benefits for the teacher are that she can assess the classes which were useful to the mothers and also allows those who are community based to have an account of recent and local hospital practice. There may be some unfavourable comment but it is unlikely as many people find it difficult to be critical of an individual in front of a group.

- *Using another teacher* – A colleague who has been part of the class or who joins by invitation can see aspects of the class that escape the one involved in teaching and can provide useful feedback.

- *Taping a class* – Try using a tape recorder in one of the classes to examine what went on. Ask the parents if they mind, assuring them it is only to improve the teaching. The aspects to listen for could include the following. Who does the most talking, the teacher or parents? What was the content, did it relate to what the parents wanted to talk about? Did the teacher ask many questions and how did the parents reply? Was it always one or two words or longer responses? Did the same person answer every time? Did one person dominate the class or was there a lot of background chatter? It can be time consuming to listen to tapes in detail but if the occasional class is taped it can help the teacher to be aware of what she is doing; see Perkins (1980a) for further details.

- *Questionnaires* – Asking those attending the classes to complete evaluation forms is another means of obtaining feedback. The teacher needs to consider if the form will be given out before or after the babies' births. The classes may be fresh in parents' minds before they go into labour but it is only postnatally that they will know whether or not the information has been useful. Questionnaires can also be used for those not attending classes to discover the reasons for low attendance; a change in the bus times may be more influential than the content or teaching of the classes.

All classes are different and there should be the possibility of constantly changing and adapting to individuals and their needs. Such an approach to teaching helps the teacher to enjoy her classes so that they do not become boring and repetitive but remain alive and vibrant.

☐ **Acknowledgements**

The study on which this chapter was based was funded by the (then) Health Education Council and academic supervision was by Ann Faulkner.

■ References

Adams L 1982 Consumers' view of antenatal education. Health Education Journal 41: 12–16

Amos A, Jones L, Martin C 1988 Maternity services in Lothian: a report on a survey of users' opinions. Maternity Services Group, Edinburgh Local Health Council, University of Edinburgh

Ashton R M 1977 The parentcraft teacher. Nursing Mirror 146 (Parentcraft Supplement): xv

Ball J A 1981 Effect of present patterns of maternity care on the emotional needs of mothers: Part 2. Midwives Chronicle 94 (1123): 198–202

Bonovich L 1981 Participation: the key to learning for patients in antepartal clinics. Journal of Obstetric, Gynecologic and Neonatal Nursing 10: 75–9

Boswell J 1979 Are classes 4 and 5 paying attention? Nursing Mirror 148 (12): 24–5

Boyd C, Sellars L 1982 The British way of birth. Pan Books, London

Brammer A C 1977 Organised classes for pregnant women and their partners in preparation for childbirth and parenthood: An enquiry into the classes provided by the Maternity Services in England in 1975. Maws Ed Research Scholarship. RCM, London

Brant H A 1978 The quality of prenatal care. Midwives Chronicle 91 (1098): 315–18

Breese A C 1976 Antenatal classes and preparation for pregnancy, birth and motherhood. Unpublished M Med Sci dissertation, University of Nottingham

Brown B 1982 Maternity-patient teaching – a nursing priority. Journal of Obstetric, Gynecologic and Neonatal Nursing 11: 11–13

Burnett C W F 1956 The value of antenatal exercises. Journal of Obstetrics and Gynaecology 63: 40–57

Burrell A H 1988 A new approach to parentcraft. Health Visitor 61: 111

Campbell A, Worthington E L 1982 Teaching expectant fathers how to be better childbirth coaches. American Journal of Maternal and Child Nursing 7: 28–32

Carey J 1981 First trimester prenatal counseling in private practice. Journal of Obstetric, Gynecologic and Neonatal Nursing 10: 336–39

Central Midwives Board 1962 Handbook incorporating the rules of the CMB. CMB, London

Central Midwives Board 1980 Approved midwifery training syllabus. CMB, London

Chamberlain G 1975 Antenatal education: the consumers' view. Midwife, Health Visitor and Community Nurse 11 (8): 289–329

Chng A, Magwene K, Frand E 1987 Increased safety belt use following education in childbirth classes. Birth 14: 148–52

Cogan R 1978 Practice times in prepared childbirth. Journal of Obstetric, Gynecologic and Neonatal Nursing 7: 33–8

Cogan R, Henneborn W, Klopfer F 1976 Predictors of pain during prepared childbirth. Journal of Psychosomatic Research 20: 523–33

Craig P M 1981 Organising and co-ordinating antenatal education in preparation for parenthood. Unpublished report for Liverpool Area Health Authority (Teaching)

Craven R O, Crouch M, Goosey R A 1975 Guidelines for teachers of parentcraft and relaxation. Midwives Chronicle 88 (8 parts): 11–12; 55; 84–5: 118; 155; 205; 236; 266–67

DHSS 1976 The future role of the midwife in the maternity services. Discussion paper Annex to CNO (7c): 20

Draper J, Field S, Thomas H, Hare M J 1982 The level of preparedness for parenthood. Maternal and Child Health 7: 44–7

Enkin M 1982 Antenatal classes. In Enkin M, Chalmers I (eds) Effectiveness and satisfaction in antenatal care. Spastics International Medical Publications. Heinemann, London

Farleys Report 1988 Is having babies the end of life as we know it? Crookes Healthcare

Genest M 1981 Preparation for childbirth – a review. Journal of Obstetric, Gynecologic and Neonatal Nursing 12: 82–5

Giefer M A, Nelson C 1981 A method to help new fathers develop parenting skills. Journal of Obstetric, Gynecologic and Neonatal Nursing 12: 455–57

Gillett J 1976 A report on the survey on preparation for childbirth within the catchment area of Copthorne Maternity Unit, Shrewsbury. International Journal of Nursing Studies 13: 25–46

Greenberg J S, Sullivan R 1977 The need for prenatal health education. Health Education Journal 36: 84–7

Greenwood J 1983 Whose baby? Midwives Chronicle 96 (1150): 334–38

Griffiths C S, Jenner A M 1985 An evaluation of dental health education for parentcraft groups. Health Education Journal 44: 120–23

Heardman M 1982 Relaxation and exercise for childbirth (5th ed). Churchill Livingstone, Edinburgh

Hibbard B M, Robinson J O, Pearson J F, Rosen M, Taylor A 1979 The effectiveness of antenatal education. Health Education Journal 38: 39–46

Homans H Y 1980 Pregnant in Britain: a sociological approach to Asian and British women's experiences. Unpublished PhD thesis, University of Warwick

Husband L 1983 Antenatal education: its use and effectiveness. Health Visitor 56: 409–10

Jacoby A 1988 Mothers' views about information and advice in pregnancy and childbirth: findings from a national study. Midwifery 4: 103–10

Jamieson L 1981 Education means teamwork. Nursing Focus 3: 260–3

Jamieson L 1982 Paper for the Health Education Council. Unpublished

Jamieson L 1986 Education for parenthood. Nursing 3: 13–16

Jiminez S L M 1980 Education for the childbearing year: comprehensive application of psychoprophylaxis Journal of Obstetric, Gynecologic and Neonatal Nursing 11: 97–9

Jukes K 1988 Antenatal lucky bag. New Generation (March): 37

Kitzinger S 1972 The experience of childbirth (3rd ed). Penguin Books, Harmondsworth

Kuczynski H J 1984 Benefits of childbirth education – the first stage of life. Midwives Chronicle 97 (1158): 188–92

Kuczynski H J, Thompson L 1985 Be prepared. Nursing Mirror 16 (10): 26–8

Laughran M 1973 A project on antenatal health education in Manchester. Midwife and Health Visitor 9: 195–97

McCabe F, Rocheron Y, Dickson R, McCron R 1984 Antenatal education in primary care: a survey of general practitioners, midwives and health visitors. Centre for Mass Communication Research, University of Leicester (1984)

McIntosh J 1988 A consumer view of birth preparation classes: attitudes of a sample of working class primiparae. Midwives Chronicle 101 (1199): 8–9

McKenna J 1976 Antenatal preparation and epidural anaesthesia. Midwife, Health Visitor and Community Nurse 12 (2): 78–80

Mandlestram D A 1971 The value of antenatal preparation – a statistical survey. Midwife and Health Visitor 7 (5): 217–24

Morgan J 1984 Effect of antenatal education on expectant parents' knowledge and attitudes regarding infant nutrition. Health Education Journal 43: 104–7

Myles M F 1975 Textbook for midwives (8th ed). Churchill Livingstone, Edinburgh

Murphy-Black T 1986 Evaluation of a post basic training course for teachers. Unpublished PhD thesis, University of Manchester

Murphy-Black T, Faulkner A 1987 Antenatal groups skills training: a manual of guidelines. John Wiley, Chichester

Newson J, Newson E 1965 Patterns of infant care in an urban community. Pelican Books, Harmondsworth

Niven C 1984 Labour pain. Research and the Midwife Conference Proceedings. King's College, University of London

Oakley A 1981 Adjustment of women to motherhood. Nursing 1 (21): 899–901

O'Brien M, Smith C 1981 Women's views and experiences of antenatal care. The Practitioner 225: 123–25

Orr J 1980 Health visiting in focus. RCN, London

Perkins E R 1978a Having a baby: an educational experience? Leverhulme Health Education Project Occasional Paper No 6, University of Nottingham

Perkins E R 1978b Antenatal classes in Nottinghamshire, the pattern of official provision. Leverhulm Health Education Project Occasional Paper No 9, University of Nottingham

Perkins E R 1978c Attendance at antenatal classes: a district study. Leverhulme Health Education Project Occasional Paper No 13, University of Nottingham

Perkins E R 1978d And did you go to classes, Mrs Brown? Midwives Chronicle 92 (1104): 422–25

Perkins E R 1980a Education for childbirth and parenthood. Croom Helm, London

Perkins E R 1980b Men on the labour ward. Leverhulme Health Education Project Occasional Paper No 22, University of Nottingham

Perkins E R 1981 Evaluating in service training: a practical approach. Nottingham Practical Papers in Health Education No 3, University of Nottingham

Rathbone B 1973 Focus on new mothers: a study of antenatal classes. RCN, London

Rees C 1982 Antenatal classes: time for a new approach. Nursing Times 78 (48): 1446–48

Ritchie J E 1970 The fathers' role in family centred childbirth. Midwife and Health Visitor 6 (7): 302–07

Roberts H, Wotten, I D P, Kane K M, Harnett W E 1953 The value of antenatal preparation. Journal of Obstetrics and Gynaecology of the British Empire   60: 404–08

Roberts J E 1976 Priorities in prenatal education. Journal of Obstetric, Gynecologic and Neonatal Nursing   84: 17–20

Robinson S, Golden J, Bradley S 1983 The role and responsibilities of the midwife. NERU Report No 1. Chelsea College, University of London

Rodway H E 1947 A statistical study on the effects of exercise for childbearing. Journal of Obstetrics and Gynaecology of the British Empire   54: 77–85

Royal College of Midwives 1966 Statement of policy on the maternity services. RCM, London

Sayle D M 1979 Preparing the midwife for the 1980s – is safety enough? Midwives Chronicle   92 (1100): 306–09

Skelton I 1984 Acupuncture in labour. Research and the Midwife Conference Proceedings. King's College, University of London

Sweet B 1984 Midwives in clinical practice. Nursing Times   80 (22): 60–2

Taylor A 1985 Antenatal classes and the consumer: mothers' and fathers' views. Health Education Journal   44: 79–82

Thomson A M 1980 Planned or unplanned? Are midwives ready for the 1980s? Midwives Chronicle   93 (1106): 68–72

United Kingdom Central Council 1986 Handbook of Midwives Rules. UKCC, London

Watson M, Morrison E M 1979 Health education and infant feeding – does mother know best? Midwives Chronicle   92 (1097): 220–21

Whitley N 1979 A comparison of prepared childbirth couples and conventional prenatal class couples. Journal of Obstetric, Gynecologic and Neonatal Nursing   8: 109–11

Williams M, Booth D 1974 Antenatal education guidelines for teachers. Churchill Livingstone, Edinburgh

Williamson J A 1975 Hypnosis in obstetrics. Nursing Times   71 (48): 1895–97

Willmuth R, Weaver L, Borenstein J 1978 Satisfaction with prepared childbirth and locus of control. Journal of Obstetric, Gynecologic and Neonatal Nursing   5: 33–7

Winkler E 1988 Great expectations. Parents   147: 87–8

Worthington E L, Martin G A, Shumate M 1982 Which prepared-childbirth coping strategies are effective? Journal of Obstetric, Gynecologic and Neonatal Nursing   11: 45–51

Zacharias J F 1981 Childbirth education classes: effects on attitudes toward childbirth in high risk indigent women. Journal of Obstetric, Gynecologic and Neonatal Nursing   10: 165–67

Zax M, Sameroff A J, Farnum J E 1975 Childbirth education, maternal attitudes and delivery. American Journal of Obstetrics and Gynecology   123: 185–90

■ Suggested further reading

Kitzinger S 1977 Education and counselling for childbirth. Baillière Tindall, London

Murphy-Black T, Faulkner A 1987 Antenatal groups skills training: a manual of guidelines. John Wiley, Chichester

Perkins E R 1980 Education for childbirth and parenthood. Croom Helm, London

Williams M, Booth D 1983 Antenatal education guidelines for teachers. Churchill Livingstone, Edinburgh

Chapter 7

Ultrasound – the midwife's role

Jean Proud

Ultrasound scanning of the pregnant uterus is considered by many to have become an important part of antenatal care. Most women expect it to be performed, and many feel deprived if it is not offered. The policy of many obstetricians is to 'scan' women routinely between 18 and 20 weeks gestation when the fetus is easily visualised. The uterus is then an abdominal organ and the fetus is sufficiently large for all the major systems to be examined for any defects. It is sufficiently early in the pregnancy to give an accurate estimation of gestational age and not too late to eliminate the possiblity of multiple pregnancy, or the presence of an extra abdominal mass.

An ultrasound scan may be performed earlier in pregnancy to:

- Confirm pregnancy and establish gestional age at the first clinic visit;

- Confirm or exclude an extra-uterine pregnancy;

- Confirm or exclude multiple pregnancy (see page 108);

- Investigate fetal viability;

- Confirm or exclude the presence of an associated abdominal mass;

- Diagnose hydatidiform mole.

Scans may be performed later in pregnancy for a variety of reasons – for instance, to locate a placenta following antepartum haemorrhage or as a screening test to detect intra-uterine growth retardation.

Although ultrasound is of undoubted value in the management of some pregnancies, it is sometimes misused. Ultrasound scans cannot provide a solution to every diagnostic problem and in some instances other resources may be more appropriately used. Conversely, the full potential of ultrasound may not always be realised.

This chapter will address the indications for, and safety of, ultrasound scanning (USS) in pregnancy, and the role of scanning personnel, particularly that of the 'scanning midwife'

■ It is assumed that you are already aware of the following:

- What ultrasound is and how it works;
- The development and use of ultrasound in pregnancy and the postnatal period;
- Indications for the use of diagnostic ultrasound in pregnancy and postnatally.

■ The major uses of ultrasound scanning in pregnancy

□ Assessment of gestational age

For some time ultrasound scanning has been widely used to assess gestational age with accuracy. The value of this has become clear in an age when the combined oral contraceptive pill is popular, or when women cannot recall the date of their last menstrual period. The usual method of estimating an expected date of delivery (EDD) is by applying Naegele's rule. This calculates the EDD from the first day of the last menstrual period and so of course may only be used when the woman can give an accurate account of her menstrual history. The use of a combined oral contraceptive or the presence of bleeding in early pregnancy may limit the use of this method. Studies investigating the use of Naegele's rule (Campbell 1974; Grennert *et al* 1978; Bennett *et al* 1982) indicate that between 6 per cent and 45 per cent of women are unable for various reasons to provide reliable menstrual histories, so an ultrasound scan may then be needed to date the pregnancy. Many women however (particularly those who have undergone treatment for infertility) are quite able to provide an accurate menstrual history. The practice of subjecting these women to an ultrasound scan merely to confirm what is already known is questionable.

An ultrasound scan is an essential element of a maternal serum alpha feto protein (AFP) screening programme as accurate estimation of gestational age eliminates much of the stress resulting from raised levels of AFP due entirely to wrong dating.

Diagnosis of intra-uterine growth retardation is difficult when no early 'dating' scan has been performed.

The estimation of gestational age is most accurate before 24–28 weeks of pregnancy. In the third trimester, fetal growth is relatively slow and the normal parameters of growth consequently become wider, making the accurate dating of pregnancy almost impossible (Hadlock *et al* 1982a). Measurements in frequent use include crown rump length (CRL) which represents the length of the embryo from the top of its head to its rump. This is the only practical way of measuring a tiny embryo and is used until approximately 12 weeks gestation. A more accurate measurement is the bi-parietal diameter (BPD) which can be performed in the second and third trimesters (Warsof *et al* 1983). This diameter is measured between the two parietal eminences of the fetal skull. The length of a limb (usually the femur – FL) can be measured and in conjunction with the BPD is the usual method of assessing gestational age in the second trimester. The head circumference (HC) is also used in the assessment of gestational age. The abdominal circumference (AC), measured at the level of the bifurcation of the main portal vein into its right and left branches, can be used in conjunction with other measurements as a prediction of gestational age. Because of biological variability and inaccuracies of measurement, this is a poor parameter on its own (Hadlock *et al* 1982b). The abdominal area can be assessed at the same level and is preferred by some operators as it is said to be a more accurate measurement, however these two measurements are more often used in screening for intra-uterine growth retardation and are not particularly useful in the assessment of gestational age.

□ **Prenatal diagnosis of fetal abnormality**

Many obstetricians consider that every pregnant woman should be offered an ultrasound scan to screen for possible fetal anomalies. In 1983, Professor Stuart Campbell advocated a detailed assessment of the following:

- Measurements of the BPD, HC, AC and FL;
- Ventricular-hemispherical ratios in the head (both anterior and posterior), examination of the cerebellum, palate, face and neck;
- Spine to eliminate neural tube defects;
- Heart to confirm the presence of four chambers, an intact ventricular septum and to exclude any major defects;
- Diaphragm to exclude the presence of any hernias;
- Abdominal wall to exclude exomphalus or a gastroschisis;
- Liver, umbilical vein, exclusion of abdominal masses;
- Kidneys, structure and size of renal pelvis;

- Limbs, fingers and toes to exclude achondroplasia, osteogenesis imperfecta and/or any possible amputations or abnormal limb growth;

- Placental structure and amniotic fluid volume;

- Number of vessels in the umbilical cord;

- In units with the necessary additional equipment, uterine and fetal blood flow measurements can be taken at this time. Changes in the uteroplacental circulation in the form of increased waveforms are said to indicate a pregnancy that is 'at risk'. Abnormal waveforms are said to be associated with a high incidence of intra-uterine growth retardation and fetal asphyxia (Pearce 1987).

If anomalies are discovered early enough there is time to discuss with the parents, paediatricians, geneticists and any other relevant personnel the course of further action – for instance, transfer of the woman to the most advantageous centre for delivery, therapeutic procedures *in utero* or termination of pregnancy. One must, however, be aware of the possibility of mistaken diagnosis which could lead to termination of pregnancy being carried out when the fetus is normal. During ultrasound investigations and other screening procedures performed in the antenatal period (for example the maternal serum alpha feto protein programme), parents are subjected to a great deal of stress. Midwives will be aware of the need of many couples in such circumstances for counselling and support (Kenyon 1988).

☐ Diagnosis of a multiple pregnancy

Clinical diagnosis of a multiple pregnancy is not always reliable (Hawnylyshyn *et al* 1982). The perinatal mortality rate has not improved over recent years at the same rate as that in singleton pregnancies (Centrulo *et al* 1980; MacGillivray 1980). Early diagnosis of a multiple pregnancy facilitates close monitoring of fetal growth and wellbeing. A study carried out in Sweden (Grennert *et al* 1978) found that early diagnosis of multiple pregnancy by ultrasound examination improved the perinatal mortality rate of twins. There was a significant decrease in the preterm delivery rate and an increase in birthweight in the group of twins who had been diagnosed before the third trimester.

It is difficult, however, to establish what constitutes growth retardation in twin pregnancies and very few studies have been done to establish normal growth patterns. Socal *et al* (1984) and Secker *et al* (1985) suggested that there was a normal slowing of growth in the third trimester in twin pregnancies, so that special charts need to be constructed for use in monitoring twin pregnancies.

For more details about twin pregnancies, and in particular about the midwife's role at the time of diagnosis, the reader is referred to Chapter 9 in this volume, 'Multiple births – parents' anxieties and the realities'.

☐ Localisation of the placenta

Since ultrasound became available it has been used widely to locate the placenta following antepartum haemorrhage, in an abnormal lie, or high presenting part at term. On occasions, the presence of a retroplacental clot can be seen in cases of placental abruption. It has been observed (Gottesfield *et al* 1966; Rizos, 1979) that 20–30 per cent of women have a low lying placenta in early pregnancy, but as the uterus grows and the lower segment develops, the placental edge moves progressively further away from the internal os. Approximately 5 per cent of women who present with a low lying placenta in the second trimester have a true placenta praevia at term (Gottesfield *et al* 1966; Rizos 1979).

☐ The textural appearance of the placenta

The textural appearance of the placenta alters with advancing gestation (Grannum *et al* 1979). From 1983–6 a randomised controlled trial (Proud 1987) was conducted at a district hospital to test, firstly, the hypothesis that early placental maturation is a predictor of subsequent obstetric problems and, secondly, whether clinical action taken on the basis of placental grading improves perinatal outcome. Two thousand women were studied. An observational study was also done on the 1468 women who were scanned between 34–36 weeks gestation. An association was found between early placental maturation and maternal smoking. Two hundred and twenty-three of the 1468 were found to have a mature placenta at this scan; of these 83 (37 per cent) admitted to smoking when they were interviewed at booking. Of the remaining 1245 women whose placentae had a normal appearance for that gestation, only 23 per cent admitted to smoking. Other associations with an early maturing placenta were:

- Meconium staining of the liquor (p value < 0.001);

- Emergency caesarean section for fetal distress ($p < 0.005$);

- Apgar score <7 at five minutes after birth ($p < 0.05$);

- Low birth weight ($p < 0.025$);

- Perinatal death ($p < 0.005$).

More detail of the exact numbers and percentages involved is given in Table 7.1.

Table 7.1 Early placental maturation and subsequent obstetric problems

	Placental grade	
	0–2	3
Meconium staining	no: 1245	no: 223
	7%	14%
Emergency caesarean section for fetal distress	no: 1256	no: 227
	2%	6%
Apgar score < 7 at 5 mins	no: 1256	no: 227
	1.3%	3.1%
Low birthweight	no: 1256	no: 227
	5.5%	10.6%
Perinatal death	no: 1256	no: 227
	0.24%	1.76%

Source: Proud 1987

For the second part of the study, the 2000 subjects were divided into two groups. Randomisation produced groups that were compatible in all aspects. In the first group placental grading was reported to the obstetricians for all ultrasound examinations. In the second group the placenta was graded, but this grading was recorded only for the purposes of the study and was not reported to the clinicians.

Changes in the management in the 'revealed' group were few. The main response to the report of early placental maturation seems to have been oestriol estimation ($p < 0.01$). There were slightly fewer inductions, 218 to 237 in the concealed group, but 59 elective lower segment caesarean sections to 55 in the concealed group. There was a difference in perinatal deaths between the groups, there being two in the revealed group and ten in the 'concealed' group not associated with lethal malformations.

The results of the study, confirmed the associations between early maturation of the placenta and problems in labour, poor condition at birth, and low birth weight. None of the sensitivities were particularly high, with the possible exception of normally formed stillbirths ($p < 0.05$). Chances of subsequent obstetric problems are apparently more than doubled in association with early placental maturation, but actual problems are likely to develop in only a few of these cases. This suggests that finding a mature placenta at 34–36 weeks gestation should lead to increased surveillance and supplementary tests of fetal wellbeing rather than more definitive obstetric intervention. It was therefore recommended that grading a placenta be one of the indices reported during ultrasound examination in the third trimester.

☐ Diagnosis of intrauterine growth retardation

Until recently it has been standard practice in many maternity units to use ultrasound to screen routinely for intrauterine growth retardation. Poor fetal growth has long been accepted as a major factor associated with perinatal mortality and morbidity. Measurement of the head alone by the BPD or head circumference is insufficient due to the fact that in many instances the brain is 'spared' in a fetus suffering from this condition. Liver size is reduced, however, so an abdominal circumference should be a more sensitive parameter. A comparison of the two in the form of a ratio HC/AC (Campbell 1977) is thought to be valuable.

Various other combinations of measurements have been suggested – for example, CRL – and abdominal areas (Neilson *et al* 1984) – but screening is difficult due to the wide variations in fetal growth that fall within normal limits. Any measurements should be combined with other parameters. Instead of routine ultrasound screening for intrauterine growth retardation, many maternity units have returned to using the measurement between the symphysis and fundal height by tape measure. This is very simple to perform and a prospective study at Kings College Hospital (Pearce & Campbell 1983) found it to be as efficient as ultrasound screening, both detecting about 85 per cent of cases.

Selective techniques now used in ultrasound departments for diagnosis of intrauterine growth retardation include measurement of uterine blood flow and/or fetal biophysical profile scoring. Assessing the fetus in this manner requires time and the use of the most modern equipment available. In the process of biophysical profile scoring, the fetus is assessed over a period of 30 minutes as follows, a maximum score of two being given for each parameter.

- *Fetal breathing*: at least one episode of fetal breathing lasting 30 seconds should be seen during the assessment period.

- *Gross body movement*: some body or limb movement should take place at least three times during the same period of observation.

- *Fetal tone*: some extension of limb, hand or fist should take place within this time.

- *Reactive fetal heart rate*: at least two episodes of acceleration of the fetal heart should take place.

- *Amniotic fluid volume*: there should be at least one pocket of amniotic fluid that measures over 1 cm in depth.

Low scores occurring in conjunction with oligohydramnios indicate the need for intervention (Manning *et al* 1987).

☐ **Guiding during invasive and therapeutic procedures**

Ultrasound is also used, for example, during amniocentesis and intrauterine transfusion.

☐ **Other uses**

Some units are fortunate enough to have a portable scanner or scanners. These can be particularly useful on the labour suite or in the community. Presentation can be confirmed, and estimation of gestational age assessed in the doctor's surgery or the woman's home. More sophisticated examinations, however, are best performed on machines with better resolution than portable scanners can provide.

■ The safety of ultrasound

The use of ultrasound has undoubtedly revolutionised antenatal care. Iain Donald's prophecy, made in a speech in the mid 1970s, that 'The day may come shortly when routine ultrasound examination will be offered to every pregnant patient' has been realised. Ultrasound technology has developed quickly and, until 1984 when the media suddenly brought to public attention the possibility of some possible hazard in its use for diagnostic purposes, especially to the pregnant woman, the advisability of its use was not seriously questioned.

Since the inception of ultrasound scanning in medicine in the early 1970s, investigations have been carried out to identify possible hazards associated with its use. Sound waves are partially absorbed by body tissues and in the process of this absorption a certain amount of heat is produced. Possible adverse effects of this heat production have been sought. The variation in temperature, however, has been found to be no more than that which occurs naturally in the body diurnally. Heat produced by ultrasound is therefore unlikely to cause damage.

Because sound waves vibrate, some displacement of tissue particles will occur, so it is important that intensities within the ultrasound beam are known to the operator and are kept to a minimum. Cavitation (the formation of gaseous bubbles in the tissues), or microstreaming (the movement of the liquid surrounding an oscillating bubble) have been suggested as other possible hazards of ultrasound (ter Haar *et al* 1981). The evidence is not yet conclusive that these phenomena occur at all or, if they do, that they constitute a hazard particularly at the ultrasound output levels used for diagnostic purposes.

Studies have been undertaken to investigate the biological effects of ultrasound on cells in man and animals. It is sometimes very difficult to interpret the results of studies performed. A wide variety of laboratory models are used, and many of the intensities and exposure times of ultrasound are not given. In 1970, Mackintosh and Davey published a paper suggesting that some chromosomal damage could occur as a result of ultrasound used for diagnostic purposes; however other studies published over the next few years (Hill *et al* 1972, Coakley *et al* 1972, Buckton & Baker 1972, Watts *et al* 1972) could not confirm these results. Mackintosh (1975) was himself unable to obtain the same results when repeating the original experiments. Leibskind *et al* (1979) reported an increase in sister chromatid exchanges in human lymphocytes when exposed to diagnostic ultrasound in the laboratory situation. These results however have not been confirmed in the clinical situation. Attempts have been made to simulate *in vivo* conditions by using freshly delivered placental tissue, and similar results were obtained. More recent studies (Robinson *et al* 1981; Wegner & Meyenburg 1980) have shown no genetic alterations and no increase in sister chromatid exchanges.

Other areas of investigation have included the effects of ultrasound on embryonic growth, cell surfaces, and the immunological, blood coagulation, nervous and reproductive systems. To date, no evidence has emerged to identify possible related hazards (Wells 1987a).

Epidemiological studies have involved children exposed to ultrasound *in utero*. Bernstein (1969) followed up 720 babies who had had their fetal hearts monitored *in utero* by continuous wave doppler, for auscultation purposes. Hellman *et al* (1970) collected data from three centres to examine the possible connection between ultrasound exposure during the antenatal period and subsequent fetal abnormalities. The incidence of abnormalities was 2.7 per cent in the exposed group and 4.8 per cent in the group with no ultrasound exposure. Two other research projects (Bakketeig *et al* 1984, Neilson *et al* (1984) involved randomised controlled trials, the primary aim of which was to determine the benefits of ultrasound screening in pregnancy from the point of view of clinical outcome. The evidence revealed that there were marginal benefits only, and no evidence was found of any deleterious effects due to ultasound exposure. No evidence has been found either to suggest that exposure to ultrasound *in utero* is a contributory factor in childhood malignancy; but follow up studies are still in progress.

Correlations have been sought between ultrasound and dyslexia (Stark *et al* 1984), hearing problems, neoplasms, malformations and behavioural problems (Lyons & Coggrave-Toms 1979). No statistically significant associations have been found, but in some circles it is considered that the slight increases in numbers in the exposed groups, particularly in association with dyslexia, are worrying and need further extensive study.

A working party set up in 1984 by the Diagnostic Methods Committee of the British Institute of Radiology (Wells 1987a) considered the evidence presently available for and against the use of diagnostic ultrasound. They concluded that whereas there is at the moment no evidence to suggest diagnostic ultrasound is potentially harmful, ultrasound should only be performed for a valid clinical reason and not just to 'watch the baby'. The working party stressed the need for further long term research into possible adverse effects, and in the meantime advocated constant vigilance in monitoring the safety of antenatal ultrasound scans. Recommendations were also made regarding the output of scanning machines and the training of ultrasound personnel.

In 1984 The World Health Organisation (WHO) called for more randomised controlled trials of ultrasound scanning in pregnancy. It would, however, be extremely difficult to persuade pregnant women, obstetricians, and ethical committees to participate in such trials. Many women would be denied ultrasound, when at the present time there is insufficient evidence that it is harmful. Few women would agree to forego a procedure generally considered to be part of good antenatal care. The value of ultrasound has not been confirmed however, and (bearing in mind past lessons learnt from thalidomide and the dangers of X-rays) the possible risks of ultrasound need to be acknowledged and weighed against the perceived advantages.

The Royal College of Obstetricians and Gynaecologists (RCOG 1984) has recommended that routine ultrasound examination between 16–20 weeks of pregnancy should continue as gestational age may be established, and multiple pregnancies or fetal anomalies can be diagnosed. The fetus 'at risk' can be identified and the mother offered a more intensive style of care during pregnancy which should improve the chances of a good perinatal outcome. Similarly, the 'low-risk' pregnancies may be identified and ante-natal and intrapartum care planned accordingly. Mothers in this group could perhaps be offered more community antenatal care, thus reducing the size of consultant's clinics. The consequent benefits would include shorter waiting times at clinics, less time spent travelling and more efficient use of resources.

Most pregnant women expect to have an ultrasound scan. For many, indeed, it is an integral part of having a baby. They look forward to it and so, often, do their partners. This privileged look at their baby may be anticipated by both parents with great excitement. Although this attitude is perfectly understandable, it can at times cause difficulties for the ultrasonographer who has a detailed examination to perform and a great many measurements to record in a limited time.

A degree of bonding takes place as a result of the scan. In a small study by Campbell *et al* (1982), the psychological impact of ultrasound scans upon two groups of pregnant women was examined. One group was allowed to watch the screen during the scan, the other were not. A questionnaire was given to both groups to try to assess the parental attitude to the pregnancy. The group allowed to watch the screen during the examination felt stronger emotional ties to their fetus than the group who did not.

It is desirable that the possible hazards of ultrasound, as well as its benefits, are discussed so that women are able to make an informed decision regarding whether or not to undergo the investigations. The RCOG (1984) stated that while they considered written consent unnecessary, they recommended that a written explanation of the reasons for the scan should be given to women. Scanning personnel should ensure that the content of the written explanation has been read and understood. This recommendation is consistent with the Midwives' Code of Practice and the UKCC Code of Professional Conduct. It is questionable, however, whether it is possible to follow this advice very closely in busy scanning departments. Discussions of this nature are perhaps best undertaken by the midwives in the antenatal clinic, at the time when other screening procedures are explained, thus giving time for parents to consider the implications of the scan and make their decision.

■ The prudent use of ultrasound

Following publication of the reports of the working parties at the RCOG (1984) and The British Institute of Radiology (Wells 1987a), the British Medical Ultrasound Society (BMUS) set up a working party of its own, to examine the results of the two reports and to look at the wider issue of the prudent use of diagnostic ultrasound (BMUS 1988). With this issue in mind they made certain recommendations. These were, firstly, that output levels of ultrasound advocated by the American Institute of Ultrasound in Medicine over the last decade should be adhered to. These levels provide a large safety factor between therapeutic and diagnostic levels. Secondly, the BMUS recommended that the examination itself should be done in the shortest possible time, gaining the maximum amount of information. Certain guidelines were given as to the exact amount of time an examination should take. This has implications on the presence of visitors in the scan room as there is no doubt that the presence of spectators distracts the operator and therefore lengthens the time needed for the examination. For instance, a great deal of concentration is required to examine a tiny fetus for abnormalities. Questions, or even expressions of delight, may interrupt such procedures. Many operators find it difficult to point out features of the scan to mothers, while at the same time conducting their investigations. Furthermore if abnormalities are discovered it can be very difficult to counsel parents if other members of the immediate or the extended family are present. For these reasons, many units restrict the number of people allowed into the scan room; some units prefer even the father to remain outside, at least until the detailed measurements have been recorded.

The BMUS also made recommendations regarding the training of ultrasonographers, from all disciplines. They advocated that there should be standard methods of assessment and accreditation. They recommended ways in which ultrasonographers should keep up to date with advancing techniques and the need for refresher courses at frequent intervals. They also emphasised the premise that there is no place for the trivial scan.

Professor Peter Wells (1987b) in his presidential address to the British Institute of Radiology took this subject as his theme. He said 'The prudent use of ultrasound diagnosis depends on it being used cautiously, carefully, circumspectly, judiciously, sensibly and wisely. Like other technologies in medicine diagnostic ultrasound is a resource which should be used with skill and good judgement'.

■ Recommendations for clinical practice in the light of currently available evidence

Although several issues identified below would appear to relate primarily to midwives performing ultrasound scans, this section asks questions that should be considered by all midwives since scanning may be perceived as a possible extension of the role of the midwife.

Midwives performing ultrasonography should consider carefully the issues involved in their particular working environment in the light of the Midwives' Code of Practice (1989) and the UKCC Code of Professional Conduct (1985). These are some of the questions that need to be addressed:

1. Is 'routine' ultrasound scanning practised in your department? In your opinion, is it justifiable? If not, what action (if any) should you take?

2. What course of action do you take when a scan is requested for no apparent good clinical reason?

3. Are there circumstances when you would refuse to perform an ultrasound scan when it has been requested by the clinician?

4. Has your training fully equipped you to use this technology and to interpret the results? If it has not, what action should you take?

5. Should midwives be scanning at the level of detailed fetal anatomical surveys? If you do, what supervision and support do you expect and receive? From whom do you receive it?

6. Are you scanning in situations where there is no obstetrician or radiologist with obstetric ultrasound scanning expertise? If so, what happens if you make a mistake? In such circumstances what is your professional, legal and ethical position?

7. Should scanning be considered as an 'extended' role for midwives?

8. Bearing in mind all these questions, should midwives be performing ultrasound scans?

■ Practice check

Although few midwives actually perform scans, most midwives are involved with women during their antenatal period. The following issues are therefore pertinent to all.

- Do the women in your care fully understand the reasons for their scan?
- Have they had ample opportunty to ask questions and/or refuse the investigation if they wish?
- Are scrupulous records kept of each scan performed?

Midwives have a duty to keep abreast of research into ultrasound, particularly with regard to its safety. As Iain Donald, speaking to ultrasound operators in 1976, said: 'Those of us who are users in clinical practice carry the main onus of responsibility for satisfying not only ourselves but the world at large that our techniques are safe.'

■ References

Bakketeig L, Eik-nes S H, Jacobsen G, Ulstein M K, Brodtkorb C J, Balstad P, Eriksen B C, Jorgensen N P 1984 Randomised controlled trial of ultrasonographic screening in pregnancy. Lancet   ii: 207–11

Bennett M J, Little G, Dewhurst C J, Chamberlain G 1982 Predictive value of ultrasound measurement in early pregnancy: a randomised controlled trial. British Journal of Obstetrics and Gynaecology   89: 338–41

Bernstein R L 1969 Safety studies with ultrasonic doppler technique. Obstetrics and Gynaecology   34: 707–09

British Medical Ultrasound Society 1988 Report of a working party on the prudent use of diagnostic ultrasound. BMUS, London

Buckton K E, Baker N V 1972 An investigation into possible chromosome damaging effects of ultrasound on human blood cells. British Journal of Radiology   45: 340–42

Campbell S 1974 The assessment of fetal development by diagnostic ultrasound. British Journal of Obstetrics and Gynaecology   75: 568–71

Campbell S, Pearce M J 1983 The prenatal diagnosis of fetal structural anomalies by ultrasound. Clinics in Obstetrics and Gynaecology   10: 475–507

Campbell S, Reading A E, Cox D N, *et al* 1982 Short term psychological effects of early ultrasonic scanning in pregnancy. Journal of Psychosomatic Obstetrics and Gynaecology   1: 57–62

Campbell S, Thoms A 1977 Ultrasound measurement of the fetal head to abdominal circumference ratio in the assessment of growth retardation. British Journal of Obstetrics and Gynaecology   84: 165–74

Centrulo C L, Ingardia C J, Sbarra A J 1980 Management of multiple gestation. Clinical Obstetrics and Gynaecology   23: 533–41

Coakley W T, Slade J S, Braeman J M 1972 The examination of lymphocytes for chromosome aberrations after ultrasonic irradiation. British Journal of Radiology   45: 328–32

Gottesfield K R, Thompson H E, Holmes J H, Taylor E S 1966 Ultrasonic placentography: a new method for placental localisation. American Journal of Obstetrics and Gynecology 96: 538–47

Grannum P A T, Berkowitz R L, Hobbins J C 1979 The ultrasonic changes in the maturing placenta and their relation to fetal pulmonic maturity. American Journal of Obstetrics and Gynecology 133: 915–22

Grennert L, Pearson P H, Gennser G 1978 Benefits of ultrasound screening of a pregnant population. Acta Obstetrica et Gynaecologica Scandinavia 78 (supplement): 5–14

Hadlock F P, Deter R L, Carpenter R J, Park S K 1982a Fetal biparietal diameter: a critical re-evaluation of the relation to menstrual age by means of real time ultrasound. Journal of Ultrasound in Medicine 1: 97

Hadlock F P, Deter R L, Harris R B, Park S K 1982b Fetal abdominal circumference as a predictor of menstrual age. American Journal of Radiology 139: 367

Hawnylyshyn P A, Bartin M, Bernstein A, Papsin F R 1982 Twin pregnancies: a continuing perinatal challenge. Obstetrics and Gynaecology 59: 463–71

Hellman L M, Dufus G M, Donald I, Sunden R 1970 Safety of diagnostic ultrasound in obstetrics. Lancet i: 1133–5

Hill C R, Joshi G P, Revell S H 1972 A search for chromosome damage following exposure of Chinese hamster cells to high intensity pulsed ultrasound. British Journal of Radiology 45: 333

Kenyon S 1988 Support after termination for fetal abnormality. Midwives Chronicle 101 (1205): 190–91

Leibskind D, Bases R, Mendez F, Elequin F, Koenigsberg M 1979 Sister chromatid exchanges in human lymphocytes after exposure to diagnostic ultasound. Science 205: 1273–75

Lyons E A, Coggrave-Toms M 1979 Long term follow up study of children exposed to ultrasound in utero. In Proceedings of the 24th Annual meeting of the American Institute of Medicine: 112, Montreal

MacGillivray I 1980 Twins and other multiple deliveries. Clinics in Obstetrics and Gynaecology 7 (3): 581–600

MacIntosh I J C, Brown R C, Coakley W T 1975 Ultrasound (in vitro chromosome aberrations). British Journal of Radiology 48: 230–32

MacIntosh I J C, Davey D A 1970 Chromosome abberations induced by an ultrasonic fetal pulse detector. British Medical Journal 4: 92–3

Manning F A, Menticoglou S, Harman C R, Morrison I, Lange I R 1987 Antepartum fetal risk assessment: the role of the fetal biophysical profile score. In Fetal monitoring. Clinical Obstetrics and Gynaecology 1: 55–72

Neilson J P, Munjanja S P, Whitfield C R 1984 Screening for small for dates fetuses: a controlled trial. British Medical Journal 289: 1179–82

Neilson J P, Whitfield C R, Aitchison T C 1980 Screening for the small for dates fetus; a two stage procedure. British Medical Journal 1: 1203–06

Pearce J M 1987 Uteroplacental and fetal blood flow. In Fetal monitoring. Clinical Obstetrics and Gynaecology 1 (1): 157–84

Pearce J M, Campbell S 1983 Ultrasonic monitoring of normal and abnormal fetal growth. In Laurenson N R (ed) Principals and modern management of high risk pregnancy: 57–100. Plenum, New York

Proud J R, Grant A 1987 Third trimester placental grading by ultrasonography as a test of fetal wellbeing. British Medical Journal 294: 1641–44

Rizos N, Doran T A, Miskin M, *et al* 1979 Natural history of placenta praevia ascertained by diagnostic ultrasound. American Journal of Obstetrics and Gynecology 133: 287–91

Robinson D E, Mitchel A D, Edmunds P D 1981 Proceedings of 26th Annual Meeting of AIUM, Paper 1707. AIUM, Bethesda, MD: 122

Royal College of Obstetricians and Gynaecologists 1984 Annual meeting of the American Institute of Medicine, Montreal: 112. Report of the RCOG working party on routine ultrasound examination in pregnancy. RCOG, London

Secker N J, Kaern J, Hansen P K 1985 Intrauterine growth in twin pregnancies: prediction of fetal growth retardation. Obstetrics and Gynaecology 66: 63–8

Socal M L, Tamura R K, Sabbagha R E, Chen T, Vaisnuto N 1984 Diminished bi-parietal diameter and abdominal circumference growth in twins. Obstetrics and Gynaecology 66: 63–8

Stark C R, Orleans M, Haverkamp A D, Murphy J 1984 Short and long term risks after exposure to diagnostic ultrasound in utero. Obstetrics and Gynaecology 63: 194–200

ter Haar G R, Daniels S 1981 Evidence for ultrasonically induced cavitation in vivo. Physics in Medicine and Biology 26: 1145–49

Warsof S L, Pearce M J, Campbell S 1983 The present place of routine ultrasound screening. Clinics in Obstetrics and Gynaecology 10 (3): 445–57

Watts P L, Hall A J, Fleming J E 1972 Ultrasound and chromosome damage. British Journal of Radiology 45: 335–39

Wegner R D, Obe G, Meyenburg M 1980 Human genetics. In Lerski R A, Morley P (eds) Ultrasound 82. Pergamon press, Oxford

Wells P N T (ed) 1987a The safety of diagnostic ultrasound. Report of a British Institute of Radiology working group. British Journal of Radiology, Supplement No 20

Wells P N T 1987b The prudent use of diagnostic ultrasound. Ultrasound in Medicine and Biology 13 (7): 391–400

■ Suggested further reading

Campbell S 1974 The assessment of fetal development by diagnostic ultrasound. British Journal of Obstetrics and Gynaecology 75: 568–71

Kenyon S 1988 Support after termination for fetal abnormality. Midwives Chronicle 101 (1205): 190–91

Proud J 1989 Placental grading as a test of fetal well-being. In Robinson S, Thomson A M (eds) Midwives, research and childbirth Vol 1. Chapman and Hall, London

Royal College of Obstetricians and Gynaecologists 1984 Report of the RCOG working party of routine ultrasound examination in pregnancy. RCOG, London

Wells P N T (ed) 1987 The safety of diagnostic ultrasound. Report of a British Institute of Radiology working group. British Journal of Radiology, supplement no 20

Chapter 8

The psychology of pregnancy

Joyce Prince and Margaret Adams

Physical and mental events are closely interwoven and pregnancy is a time of rapid development in both. Alterations in hormones, physical shape and growth occur at the same time as attitudes and expectations, both of the pregnant woman and of others towards her, are changing. The progress of a pregnancy is affected to some degree by the mother's remembrance of things past, by her perception of herself as a pregnant woman, by the attitude and behaviour of others towards her, and by her anticipation of the outcome of the pregnancy. These factors have, in the main, been moulded by her experience with her own parents, her family and the wider culture of which she is a part. Midwifery training and education are by tradition concerned with physical 'things' and yet sheer survival of mother and child can, in the developed countries, almost be taken for granted. There has been a great improvement over the last two decades in the recognition of psychological needs during labour and the postnatal period. The presence of fathers in the labour ward, discussion and choice of analgesia, information about the progress of labour and encouragement of the woman to maintain an active part in the delivery are no longer exceptional. Close contact between mother and baby postnatally and, indeed, involvement of the whole family are also generally encouraged. These have come about as a result of research and/or public demand. Similar advances in the antenatal period are overdue. Numerous studies show that routine antenatal care is failing in important ways to meet the needs of the people it is supposed to serve. Oakley (1984) summarises the problems identified (travel difficulties, insufficient/ inappropriate information and advice given, unnecessary waiting) in *The Captured Womb*. Gerard Vaughan, while Minister of Health, said that women found antenatal clinics badly organised, unfeeling and ineffective (*Guardian* 1981). Family happiness and the opportunity for individual members to experience emotional and social satisfaction and to achieve their intellectual potential are legitimate goals. If health service personnel

120

are to help individuals to progress towards such goals, some understanding of the thoughts, feelings, hopes and fears of their clients is essential.

■ It is assumed that you are already aware of the following:

- That the discipline of psychology deals with the experience and behaviour of humans and animals. This is an extensive field which overlaps with the subject matter of several other disciplines – for example, biology, sociology, linguistics and anthropology. Much human and animal behaviour is observable and therefore lends itself to the systematic assessment which is the *sine qua non* of a scientific subject. Our past experience and our thinking are generally private matters and require specialised techniques if they are to be directly subjected to rigorous and properly controlled examination. What people do, what they think they do, and what they say they do may not be related in any obvious or direct way.

- That there may be a dilemma in antenatal care between professional decisions based on the perceived requirement to maximise the physical safety of mother and baby, and the decisions which the parents may wish to make arising from other criteria. For example, to enhance family cohesion, the parents may be planning for the baby to be born at home with the family present. Alternatively, the mother may wish to maintain her autonomy with minimal use of drugs and other interventions. The concept of 'the locus of control' may be useful in any analysis of this dilemma. The need to maintain control over, and responsibility for, oneself is a strong one. Attempts by professionals to ignore this need, or ride roughshod over the woman's wishes, are likely to be resisted. Negotiation is likely to bring better returns than professional directives.

- That pregnancy, particularly a first pregnancy, is an important 'rite of passage'. That is, it is one of the major status changes that a woman and her partner experience. Adjustments have to be made in changing from independence to dependence, from wife to wife-and-mother, from being a partnership to being one of a triad, and so on.

■ Critical appraisal of the research literature

Research which is relevant to this chapter is derived from:

- experimental studies with animals;
- natural observations of animals and humans (ethology);

- naturally occuring experiments with humans;
- Survey material derived from questionnaire and/or interviews with women.

☐ Experimental studies with animals

An important piece of work was started in the 1950s by Harry and Margaret Harlow with rhesus monkeys (Harlow 1958). The central question they investigated was whether the affection that develops between the mother and baby rhesus monkeys stems from satisfaction of the hunger drive or from the comfort provided by warmth and contact. In mammals the two normally occur simultaneously. They separated the two possible sources of satisfaction by providing 'model' mothers; wire models provided food and warmth, towelling models provided comfort. The results left no doubt whatever that the contact comfort generated affectional responses in the young and it was to these models, rather than to those providing food, that the babies ran at moments of insecurity and anxiety. 'The unimportant or non-existent role of the breast and act of nursing in the formation of an infant's love for its mother' (Harlow 1958) was clearly demonstrated. The value of the work to the present purpose however emerged rather later, when the babies which had been reared in these conditions grew up. They were difficult to mate and those females who did become pregnant and produced offspring seemed to have little idea of how to care for their young, who were neglected and maltreated (Harlow 1965; Seay *et al* 1964). As infants these parents had been fed and comforted with mechanical models and lacked the responsive social interaction of a normal parent-child relationship.

Normal mating and parenting behaviour was gravely disrupted in another animal experiment by Calhoun (1962). He maintained a group of rats in physically restricted conditions. They continued to reproduce but normal behaviour patterns gave place to a high level of aggression, distorted mating behaviour and neglect and maltreatment of the young such as would be incompatible with survival of the species. Rutter and Madge (1976) point out that in human affairs personal overcrowding in the home is usually more important than the population density of a particular geographical area.

The findings of these studies concur in demonstrating the vulnerability of the cycle of reproduction to environmental and social conditions.

☐ Natural observations of the behaviour of animals and humans

Ethologists have developed techniques for observing and recording behaviour which occurs naturally in the normal habitat. Such studies have added to our understanding of long sequences of apparently instinctive behaviour, of which there are many in the reproductive cycle: courtship, nesting, interaction of mother and infant immediately after birth, feeding and so on. Having charted the normal pattern of behaviour and its 'triggers' it is possible then to interfere or change the triggers to observe the effect of external stimuli on what has traditionally been considered 'instinctive' behaviour. Complex patterns of activity, essential for the survival of the species can be distorted or destroyed.

Ethological studies have been carried out with human mothers in the postnatal period (Klaus & Kennell 1970; McFarlane 1977). Mothers were left alone with their babies as soon as was practicable after birth. Babies in the Klaus and Kennell study were naked, those in McFarlane's study were wrapped. Both were filmed. The subsequent 'getting-to-know-you' activity followed a fairly orderly and predictable pattern in which the mother explored the child with her hands and eyes, gradually bringing their positions into alignment so that they were looking into each other's eyes. Most mothers also talked to their babies.

The results of these studies added to the concern about hospital policies which separated mothers and infants. There is room for work of a similar kind in the antenatal period. Most, if not all, mammals make a home or bed for their young as a prelude to delivery. The precursor to the human delivery, however, is removal from home to a foreign environment (a state of affairs in which some mammals destroy their young). We need to know more about the parameters of this removal, whether it does distort subsequent relationships, and if so whether there are ways of ameliorating or avoiding difficulties.

□ **Naturally occurring 'human experiments'**

Some mammals, if separated from their parents while still infants, are unable to parent their own offspring adequately (see above). Frommer and O'Shea (1973a, 1973b) identified a group of women in a hospital antenatal clinic who said that they had been separated from either or both parents before they were 11 years old. They were matched for age and social class with a group of women who had not had this experience. Both groups were interviewed when their babies were two to three months old, six to seven months, nine to ten months, and again when the babies reached 13 months. There was considerable overlap between the two groups though in the group who had experienced separation as children, there were more babies with feeding problems (55 per cent as compared with 23 per cent). There were also more marital problems in this group. It is not clear whether the marital and child management problems both stemmed from the childhood separation, or whether one was influencing the other. This study depends on retrospective data; as the human memory is notoriously unreliable (Bartlett

1932) corroboration of the extent and cause of the separation would be valuable. Parental death in this and other studies appears to have less damaging consequences than separation arising from disturbed relationships.

Stott (1963) found a higher than expected amount of malformation and mental handicap in the children of women who had experienced the stress of housing difficulties or marital infidelity or bereavement during pregnancy. Stressful events during pregnancy have also been found to influence the onset of premature labour (Newton *et al* 1979). There is much information kept in formal records which is put to inadequate use. Properly maintained they could be a rich source of data about spontaneous occurrences (for example house-moving, unemployment, illness and accidents in the family) as well as about changes in the pregnant woman's experiences, including fatigue, mood, sleep and relationships with those close to her. The impact of such events on the progress of a human pregnancy has not been explored in any adequate way. In an article on 'Maternal smoking and low birth weight', Simpson and Armand-Smith (1986) have urged that maternal smoking be added to the Körner data set. Until professionals have more reliable information about psychosocial cause and effect during pregnancy, care and advice on these matters will continue to rest to an undesirable extent on speculation.

☐ Survey material derived from questionnaire/interview data

Animal studies are valuable in helping to tease out the various contributions to behaviour and development of specific species. Major elements under scrutiny can be kept under control; the influence of the behaviour of one generation on that of the next can be explored in animals with a short reproductive cycle; some of the ethical problems arising with human subjects (cross-breeding for example) do not exist. Humans are infinitely more complex than even their nearest primate relative and language mediates behaviour in many ways. It is impossible to extrapolate directly from animal to human affairs, although if findings from animal studies are applied with care, they may be suggestive of the background to some human problems.

Kitzinger (1987) estimates that 'the whole system of prenatal care works efficiently for only 10 per cent of women': that is, half of the 20 per cent who are at risk of an abnormal pregnancy ¬the problems of the other half only emerge during labour. It is not surprising to find that several researchers have tried to establish how satisfied women felt with care they received in the antenatal clinic. Robinson (1985) found much duplication of physical examination as between midwife and obstetrician in the antenatal clinic; despite this, however, several surveys (Cartwright 1979; MacIntyre 1981) show that clients' satisfaction with the information and advice received, as well as their 'treatment as a person', leaves much to be desired. Until health service managers take action on the resources that are evidently being wasted through unnecessary replication of physical examination, midwives could well expand their field of interest to meet some of the psychosocial needs of pregnant women more effectively.

A report by the President of the National Childbirth Trust (Hutton 1988) on the best and worst memories of pregnancy listed 'tests without explanations' and 'undiplomatic midwives' among the worst. Others were sickness, ailments and discomforts which came as a disappointment, and tiredness. The best memories include 'being someone special' 'continuity of care', 'physical well-being' and 'being aware of the baby moving and growing'.

The Committee on Child Health Services reported in 1976 that they could find little objective evidence regarding the value of 'parentcraft' classes, or even evidence that their content had been systematically constructed (HMSO 1976). Despite this criticism Black (1984) found that an inappropriately prescriptive approach continues to be used and that health educators are reluctant to experiment with teaching method and content (see also Chapter 6 in this volume, 'Antenatal education').

The Perinatal Mortality Survey using national data shows that there are huge discrepancies between different parts of the country in reproductive complications (Butler & Bonham 1963). The Office of Population Censuses and Surveys confirmed this in 1980. For example, the perinatal mortality rate in Kingston and Richmond in Surrey was 7.6 per thousand; in Walsall it was 19.2 per thousand (OPCS 1981). The perinatal mortality rate is a sensitive indicator of social and economic conditions which it is largely beyond the power of the midwife to influence directly. A midwife working in the north west of England can expect to see a higher proportion of low birth-weight babies than her colleague in the south.

A variety of studies has examined the effects of smoking, alcohol and drugs in the mother (which arise from aspects of maternal behaviour) on the developing fetus. As long ago as 1935, Sontag and Wallace explored the effect on the fetal heart rate of cigarette smoking and vibration to the mother's abdominal wall (Sontag & Wallace 1935a, 1935b). Both induced a physiological reaction in the fetus with a demonstrable change in the fetal heart rate. Butler and Goldstein (1973) have shown that intrauterine growth is impaired by maternal smoking and that intellectual development continues to be depressed at least until the child is seven. Maternal alcohol consumption in anything but the mildest form increases the risk of miscarriage (Kline 1980) or impaired intrauterine growth (Sokol 1980). Heavy alcohol consumption may lead to fetal alcohol syndrome which is associated with retarded physical and mental development (Olegard 1979); see also Chapter 5 in this volume, 'Maternal alcohol and tobacco use'.

The thalidomide disaster of the 1960s demonstrated the damaging effect of that drug on fetal development. Poland *et al* (1986) have shown that psychological, as well as physiological factors may be involved in the onset of pregnancy induced hypertension. Experiments with pregnant animals show that fear-inducing circumstances in the absence of any physical interference with the mother can have measurable effects on their offspring (Keeley 1962).

In their study of women attending antenatal clinic, Kumar and Robson (1978) found that 12 per cent were suffering with clinically diagnosable depression. They also found that there was a significantly higher incidence of depression during the first trimester in women who had had a previous pregnancy terminated. Dana Breen (1975) draws attention to two contrasting views of pregnancy. The 'hurdle' concept is held by women who regard pregnancy as a deviation from normality; once the pregnancy is over, a return to some former state will be effected. The 'development' alternative regards pregnancy as a period of maturation and change which results in a reorganisation of the personality. Breen's complex study of 50 women having their first babies showed that the best adjusted do not experience themselves as passive or even much in accord with the cultural stereotype of femininity. They perceive themselves to be in control, rather than controlled, as autonomous and able to deal constructively with problems.

■ Recommendations for clinical practice in the light of currently available evidence

There are several reasons why psychological factors in pregnancy are important:

1. The relationship between mother and baby is underway well before the baby is born. The nature and quality of this relationship will not only affect their happiness and psychological well-being, but can also affect the baby's physical growth, social and emotional adjustment and intellectual development. Consideration of the prospective mother therefore needs to extend beyond the obvious physical care which is necessary.

2. Over two thirds of neonatal deaths are associated with low birth-weight and congenital malformation (Butler & Bonham 1963), and these problems arise directly or indirectly from factors that are present before or during birth. As will be clear from the preceding section there is considerable potential for expanding the advice and support provided during the antenatal period.

3. Some prospective mothers do not present themselves for antenatal supervision. Numerous criticisms have been made of antenatal clinics and anything which is felt to be a barrier to attendance should be

scrutinised carefully. Psychological variables influence a m̸
willingness not only to keep appointments, but also to he̸
Greater psychological awareness by midwives, therefore, co̸
encourage more effective use of the services that are available, and
consequently reduce the perinatal mortality rate. Certain vulnerable
groups of women do need special consideration. These may include
very young or elderly mothers, unsupported women on their own,
diabetic or disabled women. Women from ethnic minority groups
sometimes face particular difficulties, as do women living in
overcrowded circumstances or who are the victims of violence.
Women who have experienced any form of reproductive casualty or
who have been treated for subfertility may justifiably be anxious.
There will be a small number of women who have to make a
decision about whether or not to have the pregnancy terminated.

4. A woman may occupy a variety of roles, for example employee, wife,
   neighbour or daughter. Being pregnant will alter all of these roles to
   some degree and add another as she prepares to become a mother.
   Societies vary in the value they place upon pregnancy and
   motherhood. For some it is regarded as the crowning achievement of
   a woman's existence and infertility is a curse. Most Western societies,
   however, take a more complicated view. Pregnancy and childbearing
   often mean relinquishing a job with a consequent reduction in social
   contacts and income. This can increase the woman's dependence on
   her partner and alter the relationship between them.

5. A woman's idea of herself – particularly herself as a mother – is
   considerably influenced by her own experience of being mothered.
   Indeed, much of our behaviour is 'learned' from the way we have
   been treated.

6. Oakley (1975) recorded some of the hopes and fears of pregnant
   women who attended antenatal clinics. Some had considerable
   doubts about their competence to look after a new baby – or even
   the probability that they would like it. As a woman's own first baby
   is often her first experience of *any* baby, doubts about her own skill
   are only reasonable. There is scope for some experimental work
   (with careful evaluation) to establish how far parenting skills can be
   built up during pregnancy.

7. Most women can anticipate a normal delivery and a happy
   integration of the new baby into the family. A minority however will
   need extra help. Staff of an antenatal clinic are in a good position to
   make arrangements for the vulnerable to learn from more
   experienced and well-adjusted women. The learning of new skills and
   attitudes might be more effectively achieved through the success that
   a 'good' mother can demonstrate, by helping a woman to feel more

self-confident (realistic goals, generous praise at appropriate times) and by ensuring that she has a support network. This is likely to require the help and advice of other services – both statutory and voluntary.

8. In the course of this century, childbearing has become increasingly medicalised and is associated with being 'ill'. The fact that much antenatal provision is sited at a hospital reinforces the view that pregnancy is pathological. Survival of the species depends upon the ability to reproduce and, to that extent, pregnancy must have positive value. In advanced societies, however, pregnancy has become a somewhat mixed blessing in which joyful anticipation is tinged with anxiety (about how to manage when the baby arrives) and being subject to medical attention (and therefore ill). Role conflict – that uncomfortable state in which two or more sets of expectations and demands are pulling in opposite directions – often results in chronic indecision and at worst can lead to depression (Kumar & Robson 1978). There are several possibilities for role conflict: the career woman who relinquishes (even if temporarily) her job, the loving wife who has to think about a third party, the beautiful girl whose figure changes, the well organised woman whose timetable is threatened. A crisis, in which established patterns of conduct become ineffective – or less effective – seems inevitable. The crisis will be resolved with the discovery of new ways of thinking and behaving and the establishment of a more complex personality in which inner experience and external demands are integrated. It is possible that a very small proportion of women depressed antenatally will experience a serious psychiatric illness.

9. Women who are anxious or depressed in the antenatal period might benefit from supportive counselling. The midwife is well placed to help in this way, as she can help any woman come to terms with the normal demands pregnancy brings, particularly if she gives individual care as required by the terms of the midwifery process.

10. An understanding interest in the woman's individual circumstances – on her own family background, her partner's attitude to the pregnancy, her confidence about caring for the baby, the effects of this baby on other family members – are matters which will be relevant to all pregnant women. Some will have special needs and worries. The loss of a previous baby at any stage, the possibility of inheritance of a defect or marked maternal mood changes are a few examples of the almost limitless number of factors that might be causing concern. They may be well-founded, or they may not, but they should nevertheless be heard, attended to and recorded. Many women keep a series of antenatal clinic appointments without having

the opportunity to express themselves on matters which concern them. When next in the antenatal clinic, make an assessment of the amount of talking done by the professionals and the amount done by the women. Consider too who determines the content and course of the conversation.

11. The Royal College of Obstetricians and Gynaecologists (1984) estimated that 85 per cent of pregnant women had an ultrasound examination at some time during their pregnancy. The report recommends that ultrasound should not be performed against the mother's wish. In order to come to a sensible decision the mother needs to have all relevant information made available to her and to have all enquiries dealt with in a competent and sympathetic way.

12. Another investigation that may be considered necessary is amniocentesis. The implications of this are considerable. If any abnormality is revealed the question of abortion may arise. Views on this may range from the strictly scientific (which does not acknowledge the moral dimension), to the highly moral which regards the destruction of human life in any form or at any stage as anathema. Presumably any mother holding the second view would not agree to prenatal investigations of the fetus. Many people are probably somewhere between the two extremes and would be open to debate. Where an abnormality is revealed, informed counselling will be essential. Factual information – the extent of the problems observed, the risk of recurrence, the kind of baby that will be born if the pregnancy goes to term – must be made available. The opportunity for both the parents to discuss the pros and cons of all possible courses of action is vital. There have been complaints that doctors do not make themselves clear and sometimes do not listen. The midwife has an invaluable part to play if she is well informed on the relevant biological matters and can help the parents to review their own hopes and fears, and their relationship, in order to come to a decision that will be satisfactory, not only with regard to the immediate problem, but for the long term future.

13. Epidemiological studies show that with humans there is a marked relationship between socioeconomic status and obstetric problems (Butler & Alberman 1969) as well as with levels of intelligence and achievement (Vernon 1969). Newton *et al* (1979) have shown that stressful psychological events during pregnancy may precipitate premature labour, resulting in low birth-weight babies. Global efforts are being concentrated to reduce the incidence of low birth-weight and its unacceptably high mortality and handicap rate (WHO 1984). The World Health Organisation takes these rates as an 'indicator of progress to the goal of health for all by the year 2000'.

14. It has been suggested that psychosocial support of women reduces the incidence of preterm labour. A review of studies (Oakley & Rajan 1988) concludes that despite several methodological problems, the evidence for the effectiveness of intervention programmes which provide additional social support is satisfactory. The term 'social support' however needs clearer definition as Lumley (1988) comments.

15. Pasamanick and Knoblock (1966) have suggested that there is a continuum of reproductive casualty ranging from fetal loss at one end, to behaviour problems in the resulting child at the other. Adverse circumstances during the prenatal period may disadvantage the offspring behaviourally, and with an accumulation of insult, the risk to the offspring increases as it moves along the continuum (from right to left in Fig 8.1). It follows that a wide range of both physiological and psychological problems for the mother can affect the health, achievement and adjustment of the next generation. Understanding the psychological dimensions of pregnancy so as to detect the abnormal and the risky, is of key importance to the midwife.

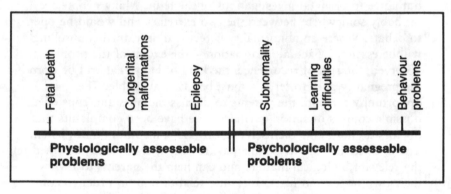

Figure 8.1   The continuum of reproductive casualty

■ Practice check

● What do you know about the family composition of women you have seen in the antenatal clinic today?

● What arrangements have been made to maximise the chances of a woman seeing the same members of staff on each antenatal visit?

● What steps do you take to give each woman the chance of asking questions, airing problems and otherwise expressing her feelings?

- What special concerns would you have for the psychological welfare of a pregnant schoolgirl?

- What information would you assemble before discussing the possibility of an abortion with a woman who has been found to be carrying a fetus with Down's syndrome? What arrangements would you make for the discussion?

- How many missed appointments are there in your antenatal clinic? What steps are you taking to improve attendance?

- Are attempts being made to resume midwives' clinics?

- Are the medical staff aware of the role of the midwife?

- Can any clinics be organised more informally and with less waiting time?

- Can clinics be arranged peripherally? Do current clinics allow time at booking for counselling when it is needed?

- Do those with special needs (for example mothers with diabetes mellitus or disabilities) have their own support group?

- Do you read the care plans in clinic before seeing each woman?

■ References

Bartlett F C 1932 Remembering. Cambridge University Press, Cambridge

Black T 1984 Antenatal education. Research and the midwife conference proceedings. London and Glasgow

Butler N R, Alberman E 1969 Perinatal problems. Livingstone, Edinburgh

Butler N R, Bonham D G 1963 Perinatal mortality: 1. Livingstone, Edinburgh

Butler N R, Goldstein H 1973 Smoking in pregnancy and subsequent child development. British Medical Journal 4: 573–75

Breen D 1975 Birth of a first child. Tavistock Publications, London

Calhoun J B 1962 Population density and social pathology. Scientific American 206: 139–48

Cartwright A 1979 The dignity of labour. Tavistock Publications, London

Frommer E A, O'Shea G 1973a Antenatal identification of women liable to have problems in managing their infants. British Journal of Psychiatry 123: 149–56

Frommer E A, O'Shea G 1973b The importance of childhood experience in relation to problems of marriage and family building. British Journal of Psychiatry 123: 157–60

Guardian 1981 New committee to fight baby deaths. 17 July

Harlow H F 1958 The nature of love. American Psychologist 12 (13): 673–85

Harlow H F 1965 Sexual behaviour in the rhesus monkey. In Beach F A (ed) Sex and behaviour. John Wiley, New York

HMSO 1976 Report of the Committee on Child Health Services. Cmnd 6684: para.8.12. HMSO, London

Hutton E 1988 The importance of the midwife: women's memories of pregnancy, labour and the postnatal period. Pregnancy: the best memories. Midwives Chronicle 10 (1207): 273–74

Keeley K 1962 Prenatal experience on behaviour of offspring of crowded mice. Science 135: 44

Kitzinger S 1987 Freedom and choice in childbirth: 105. Penguin, Harmondsworth

Klaus H M, Kennell J H 1970 Human maternal behaviour at first contact with her young. Pediatrics 46 (2): 187–92

Kline J 1980 Drinking during pregnancy and spontaneous abortion. Lancet ii: 176–80

Kumar R, Robson K 1978 Neurotic disturbance during pregnancy and the puerperium. In Sandler M (ed) Mental illness in pregnancy and the puerperium: 40–51. Oxford University Press, Oxford

Lumley J 1988 Rethinking social support in pre-term birth prevention. Birth 15 (1) 23–4

McFarlane A 1977 Psychology of childbirth: 51–4. Fontana, London

MacIntyre S 1981 Expectations and experiences of first pregnancy. Occasional Paper No. 5. Aberdeen Institute of Medical Sociology, Aberdeen

Newton R W, Webster P A C, Binu P S, Naskrey N, Phillips A B 1979 Psychosocial stress in pregnancy and its relation to the onset of premature labour. British Medical Journal 2: 411–13

Oakley A 1975 The trap of medicalized motherhood. New Society 34 (689): 639–41

Oakley A 1984 The captured womb. B H Blackwell, Oxford

Oakley A, Rajan 1988 The social support and pregnancy outcome study. Research and the midwife conference proceedings, November 1988. London and Glasgow

Office of Population Censuses and Surveys 1981 Monitor DH3 81/3 (6.10.1981). OPCS, London

Olegard R 1979 Effects on the child of alcohol abuse during pregnancy. Acta Paediatrica Scandinavica 275 (Supplement): 112–21

Pasamanick B, Knoblock H 1966 Retrospective studies on the epidemiology of reproductive casualty. Merrill Palmer Quarterly 12 (1): 7

Poland M L, Giblin P T, Lucas C P, Sokol R J 1986 Psychobiological determinants of pregnancy induced hypertension. Journal of Psychosomatic Obstetrics and Gynaecology 5: 85–99

Robinson S 1985 Responsibilities of midwives and medical staff: findings from the National Survey. Midwives Chronicle 98 (1165): 64–71

Rutter M, Madge N 1976 Cycles of disadvantage: 75. Heinemann, London

Seay B 1964 Alexander BK, Harlow HF 1964 Maternal behaviour of socially deprived monkeys. Journal of Abnormal and Social Psychology 69: 345–54

Simpson R, Armand-Smith N G 1986 Maternal smoking and low birth-weight. Journal of Epidemiology and Community Health 40: 223–7

Sokol R J 1980 Alcohol Abuse during pregnancy: an epidemiological study. Alcoholism Clinics in Experimental Research 4 (2): 135–45

Sontag L W, Wallace R F 1935a The effect of cigarette smoking during pregnancy on fetal heart rate. American Journal of Obstetrics and Gynaecology 29: 77–82

Sontag L W, Wallace R F 1935b The movement response of the human foetus to sound stimuli. Child Development   6: 253–58

Stott D H 1963 How a disturbed pregnancy can harm the child. New Scientist 320

Vernon P 1969 Intelligence and cultural environment. Methuen, London

World Health Organisation 1984. Weekly epidemiological record   59: 205

■ Suggested further reading

Breen D 1975 The birth of a first child. Tavistock Publications, London

Enkin M, Chalmers I 1982 Effectiveness and satisfaction in antenatal care: chapters 16 and 19. Spastics International, London

Kitzinger S 1987 Freedom and choice in childbirth. Penguin, Harmondsworth: chapters 1–13

Oakley A 1984 The captured womb. B H Blackwell, Oxford

Prince J, Adams M E 1987 The psychology of childbirth, 2nd ed: chapter 4. Churchill Livingstone, Edinburgh

Chapter 9

Multiple births – parents' anxieties and the realities

Jane Spillman

The revelation to parents that more than one infant has been conceived offers special opportunities for practising midwives. This chapter will explore the enhanced role of the practising midwife when caring for mothers expecting twins or a higher order multiple birth. The need for expert care is particularly pertinent at this time as *in vitro* fertilisation becomes more readily available resulting in a steadily increasing number of the higher multiples.

Multiple pregnancy is not a variant of normal pregnancy. Rather it is a high risk situation for both mother and infants which warrants particular attention.

Multiple pregnancy occurs in approximately one birth in every hundred or, to put it in another way, about one child in every fifty is one of twins. Midwives must, therefore, consider the implications of such an event for the families for whom they care. Not only is a multiple pregnancy more likely to end in spontaneous abortion, preterm delivery, fetal abnormality and perinatal bereavement, problems such as excessive morning sickness and pre-eclampsia are also more common than with singleton births (McMullan 1986a). Mothers of twins have also been shown to be more prone to atypical depression (Powell 1981).

In the past professionals tended to assume that parents would be overjoyed when told to expect more than one baby. However Spillman (1984) in a study of the effects of birthweights on mother–twin relationships has shown that this is not usually the case and that a great deal of extra support and counselling is required to prevent antenatal anxieties continuing into the postnatal period and subsequently blighting the relationships within the family.

Until recently, there were few books which addressed specific problems relating to multiple births and very little relevant research had been completed. In the last few years, however, some excellent literature, suitable both for prospective parents and for professionals and based on well-founded research, has become available. Two recent studies have looked at mothers' experiences antenatally, intrapartum and postnatally. In addition to Spillman's study described above, Barbara Broadbent (1984) compared the experiences of mothers expecting multiples at two centres in Greater Manchester with those of matched singleton mothers. These studies will be widely reported in this chapter. It is important that midwifery practice takes account of this new information to improve the prospect of a healthy outcome physically and psychologically for mothers and their 'multiple' babies.

In recent years local, national and international associations and foundations to support families with multiples have started throughout the world. Thus, the problems associated with these births and plural families have been acknowledged. Midwives should be aware of these groups and the resources which they offer.

Throughout this chapter, except where stated otherwise, the term twin includes triplets and higher order multiple births.

■ It is assumed that you are already aware of the following:

- The biology, physiology and incidence of multiple births.

- What is meant by identical and non-identical twins, usually defined as their 'zygosity'.

- Infertility and its treatment, including *in vitro* fertilisation and its implications for multiple pregnancy.

■ Multiple pregnancy is *never* planned

With modern contraceptive techniques most parents are able, if they wish, to decide when to start their families and how many children they will have. Human mothers are monotropic, that is they are conditioned to rearing only one child at a time (Bowlby 1958; Klaus & Kennell 1976; Goshen-Gottstein 1980); they never plan otherwise. This is because of the infant's long dependence on his mother. Thus it is perhaps not surprising that the reactions of parents, when given the news that more than one baby is expected, are often those of shock and disbelief (Spillman 1986). This research study resulted from a midwife's observation that mothers had special difficulties when faced with a 'plural' pregnancy which often resulted in different mothering behaviour towards each baby. Spillman (1984) studied all mothers expecting a multiple birth in the Bedford area from

Table 9.1   Anxieties expressed by mothers expecting a multiple birth

Mother worried about:	Specific examples:
1. The health of the forthcoming infants	Prematurity, low birthweight, congenital abnormality, non-survival of one or both of the twins
2. Behaviour of the babies	Sleeping patterns, feeding methods and arrangements
3. Practical worries	Coping with two or more babies, space, mobility, neglecting other duties
4. Financial considerations	Increased outlay, transport, housing, holidays etc
5. Reactions of other family members	Siblings (particularly toddlers), marital relationships, interference, criticism
6. Own health	Physical problems of multiple pregnancy, appearance, antenatal hospitalisation, difficulties of delivery, loss of identity

October 1982 to October 1983 and carried out a minimum of three tape-recorded in-depth interviews with each during pregnancy, within 48 hours of delivery and when the babies were three months old. All 27 eligible mothers were included. In addition 37 mothers who were randomly selected completed an eleven-page questionnaire covering the same aspects as the interviews. The answers of both groups were correlated and the data of all 64 participants and 128 infants was combined for analysis.

■ The diagnosis of multiple pregnancy

In times past it was quite common for mothers to learn of a multiple pregnancy shortly before or at the time of delivery. However with the advent of routine ultrasound scanning of pregnant women, it is unlikely that twins will go undetected beyond the twentieth week (Patel *et al* 1983). This is advantageous as it has been shown that early diagnosis of twins may improve the perinatal outcome (Jouppila *et al* 1985). In fact it is now possible to identify multiples in a pregnancy after only six weeks amenorrhoea (McMullan 1986a). The identification of the 'vanishing twin syndrome', where one gestational sac may disappear during the first trimester (Robinson & Caines 1977), makes it undesirable to acquaint the mother of the situation until confirmation at a later scan.

Midwives must also remember that even ultrasound may fail to detect some multiple pregnancies, and they must remain suspicious of this possibility when mothers are examined and appear larger than expected dates suggest. A recent Irish study found a 13 per cent failure rate in confirming a multiple pregnancy at the first scan (McMullan 1986b). It can be appreciated therefore, that community midwives undertaking 'shared care' of mothers must be particularly alert.

□ Reactions to the diagnosis

Spillman's research shows that the most frequent reaction of mothers to the news that more than one baby is expected is one of profound shock. Even those with a history of twins in their families do not expect it to happen to them. Some mothers report physical reactions such as sweating profusely, faintness, crying, screaming, or shaking uncontrollably. As well as disbelief, some experience anger or a feeling of isolation. A few have more positive reactions such as feeling excited, calm or euphoric but these are in the minority. Such a variety of reactions suggests that the method of telling is very important, and that a midwife or obstetrician should be available for counselling if necessary at the time or very soon afterwards (Spillman 1985).

There is a high incidence of twin pregnancy in illegitimate births, and in mothers who conceive within the first three months of marriage. Elderly mothers who already have large families are also more likely to experience a multiple pregnancy (Bulmer 1970; Eriksson & Fellman 1967). Such mothers will need special reassurance. At whatever stage the diagnosis is made and whatever the age, parity or social situation of the mother, the midwife is already likely to be involved in her care.

Ideally a midwife visiting both parents together at home as soon as possible will give the optimum support. It is important to include the father at this early stage as his role will be crucial. If he is involved in the arrangements from the beginning, he will be more prepared for the task ahead. It has also been found that mothers feel that a mother of older twins would be the person most able, after the father, to give comfort at this time (Bryan 1977; Spillman 1987b). Some hospitals offer a leaflet with contact names for the local Twins Club in the ultrasound room at the time of diagnosis, a facility that has been much appreciated (Spillman 1985).

Research has indicated that the anxieties mothers express fall into six general categories (Spillman 1984); these are listed in Table 9.1.

What then are the specific worries represented in these categories, how might they be allayed, and what are the longterm effects likely to be if they are not dealt with during the pregnancy?

☐ **The health of the forthcoming infants**

Mothers stated that preterm delivery, low birthweight, congenital abnormality and non-survival of one or both babies were particular concerns.

If one considers the possibility of such events, these anxieties would appear to be justified. Preterm delivery is quoted as high or higher than 40 per cent in some studies (Corrigan 1977; McMullan 1986b). As well as the considerable possibility of low birthweight in these preterm babies, twins and higher multiples are in any case prone to intrauterine growth retardation resulting in lower than average birthweight in the group as a whole (McMullan 1986a). When congenital anomalies are considered, there is evidence of an increased incidence of around 18 per cent (National Center for Health Statistics 1978). Perinatal mortality for twins is quoted as about four times that of singletons, for example the rate in Scotland is 53 per 1000 live births (McMullan 1986a). If triplets or higher multiples are expected, the risk is even greater.

Spillman (1984) discovered that the mothers in her study who expressed these anxieties were usually between 25 and 35 years old and and in their second or subsequent pregnancy whereas the mothers who actually experienced early delivery with its accompanying hazards tended to be either the very young mothers or those over 35 with several previous children. It is therefore possible to be reassuring in most cases.

When asked, the mothers considered below 2.5 Kg as low birthweight in the case of twin babies and 1.8 Kg in the case of triplets. Again, if such fears are expressed, reassurance that twin children reach full maturation earlier than singletons and are naturally smaller, together with information about the high survival rate and health of small babies with modern treatments may calm these fears. It is particularly counterproductive to suggest to the mother, during her pregnancy, that there may be a discrepancy between the babies' weights. This can result in the smaller baby being a focus for the mother's anxieties and in her finding great difficulty in relating to him in the early days (Spillman 1984). The effects can be long lasting. Smaller twins have been shown to exhibit frequent temper outbursts compared with their larger counterparts where mothers have stated a preference at the time of birth for the larger baby (Spillman 1987c).

If a midwife is aware of such fears, and can dispel them as soon as possible, later problems may be avoided.

☐ **The behaviour of the forthcoming babies**

The greatest concerns in this area were the likely sleeping and feeding characteristics of the twins. This was the case particularly when mothers had experienced difficulties in these aspects with previous children but even first time mothers were concerned about how they would cope. Many felt that they had received little reassurance from professionals during pregnancy. Broadbent's research (1985b) showed that mothers expecting multiples may conceal their worries or, because most of their antenatal care is at the hospital with several professionals rather than a familiar general practitioner or midwife, feel unable to ask questions or voice concerns.

Those who had the opportunity to meet other mothers of twins found this was very helpful. Once again, it would seem that the anxieties were justified. Several mothers in Spillman's study were unsuccessful with their chosen feeding methods. A recent questionnaire completed by members of the Twins and Multiple Births Association (TAMBA) into sleeping patterns in young twins found a higher incidence of problems when compared with a similar study of singletons (Edwards 1989).

☐ Practical problems

Most of the mothers wondered how they would cope with two or more babies (Spillman 1984). This was particularly true of those who were houseproud or who had several other children who needed to be taken to school, playgroups or other activities. Many were concerned about whether they would be able to get about – for example would they be able to get on to a bus with twins, a toddler and a double buggy? How would they manage to arrange two, three or more carrycots in the back of the family car? How could they possibly accommodate two drop-side cots in a tiny or already overcrowded bedroom?

☐ Financial considerations

The arrival of multiple children into a family involves considerably more financial outlay than the birth of a single child. The parents acquire an 'instant family'. Not only are two or more of everything required but nothing can be passed on from one child to another. Twin prams and buggies cost more than twice the price of the single item. If the family has been concerned about money before the pregnancy, the prospect of twins may be overwhelming. If the pregnancy was unplanned or the parents thought that their family was complete, one more baby might be absorbed but the additional costs involved in a multiple birth may produce very great stress. Often families expecting the higher multiples have found it necessary not only to change the family car to a larger one but also to move house. This of course means tremendous additional expense. Some parents feel very concerned that it will be impossible to have family outings and holidays in the future (Spillman 1986).

Many mothers expecting a multiple birth receive all or most of their antenatal care at a hospital consultant unit. The study carried out by

Broadbent in two centres in Greater Manchester (1985b) found that only 29 per cent of the mothers experienced 'shared care'. This travelling backwards and forwards to the hospital added to the expense incurred.

☐ Reactions of other family members

During pregnancy, the mothers worry a great deal about how the forthcoming infants will fit into the family. A particular concern is how siblings will react to the arrival of two or more 'competitors'. To what extent will a toddler feel 'the odd man out'? How will the older childrens' activities be fitted into a crowded schedule of feeding and changing two tiny babies?

Marital relationships are also an area of concern. If partners are not involved fully in caring for the babies, they can feel 'pushed out' as the mother strives to tackle her onerous and often overwhelming task. Sadly, marital breakdown is not uncommon in families with twins, triplets and higher multiples (Spillman 1986).

Another concern during pregnancy, is that grandparents, other relations and friends may interfere, criticise or form a preference for one of the babies. This latter point appears to reflect the mothers' own anxieties that they may feel more protective towards the smaller of twins or love one baby more than the other. Spillman's research (1984) showed that a large number of the mothers (69 per cent) did in fact form a preference in the early days. Of these over 90 per cent preferred the baby who was larger at birth. The greater the birthweight difference the more likely this was. The mothers were surprised by these reactions and felt it would have been helpful to have been warned during the pregnancy that such feelings might occur and assured this was normal. As it was, they felt extremely guilty about their reactions.

☐ Own health problems

On the whole the mothers in the study under discussion enjoyed reasonably good health during their pregnancies. They did however feel anxious about possible problems. Most ailments and discomforts associated with pregnancy in general are likely to be exacerbated when multiples are expected. Excessive and prolonged morning sickness is common and can be very tedious. Anaemia is frequently encountered. Varicose veins are a common complaint as is constipation and heartburn. Pressure on the bladder may give problems and in the later stages of the pregnancy excessive backache and difficulty in eating and sleeping may be reported (Alexander 1987).

Another problem that is common as pregnancy progresses is that of mobility. Walking can be extremely difficult. It is usual for mothers expecting a multiple birth to receive their antenatal care at a hospital

(Broadbent 1984) and this problem of mobility particularly in the later stages makes travelling to visit the hospital difficult.

Some mothers worry about their appearance as pregnancy proceeds, and may also be concerned about how their body can possibly accommodate two (or more) growing healthy babies. These women may feel extremely depressed and need much reassurance about their capacity to adapt to the situation.

Often mothers were told during their early visits to the antenatal clinic that as they were expecting more than one baby it might be necessary for them to be admitted to hospital at some stage for 'a rest'. Many of the mothers Spillman (1984) interviewed agonised over this threat throughout the pregnancy only to find that it never happened. For those who were admitted, the time in hospital appeared stressful rather than relaxing and the forthcoming babies were often blamed for the inconvenience or unhappiness. Mothers who had a toddler at home or those who had never before been separated from their partners were most upset by the hospitalisation. Recent research suggests that bedrest does not reduce the risk of preterm delivery (Koo & Green 1975; Weekes *et al* 1977; Saunders *et al* 1985).

Not surprisingly the thought of the delivery of their babies occupies the mothers' minds during the pregnancy. They may be unsure of how a delivery of more than one baby will differ, of whether their partner will be able to share the experience, of who else will be there, what equipment will be involved and whether a normal delivery is likely. These concerns are certainly justified. For example, the caesarean section rate for twin pregnancy is around double that for singletons. They are also more likely to be given epidural anaesthesia and to have a breech or forceps delivery (Broadbent 1985a). There is often a large number of people in the delivery room when twins are arriving. Most mothers accept this situation, especially if they have been warned in advance, and they may often cope better if the father is amongst those included. Spillman found that, in many cases, the mother hands over the responsibility of the first baby born to the father while the second one is arriving. When father is not there, however, the mother often cannot remember the birth of the second twin because of her concern for the firstborn (Spillman 1987a).

Monitoring equipment is likely to be used extensively during the labour of a mother giving birth to twins. Again the partner's presence can be reassuring. Men are often fascinated by technical equipment and will give encouragement to the mother to accept its use. Parents who have visited the delivery suite during the antenatal period are prepared in advance for the environment where the babies will be born and the equipment that may be used. Unfortunately unless these visits, and those to the neonatal unit are arranged at an earlier stage in the pregnancy many mothers expecting multiples never have this opportunity. They either have already delivered or are too immobile to come. In the same way, many are deprived of the relaxation and parentcraft classes which could do much to allay the problems identified by research (Spillman 1987b).

Finally some women feel that, when they face the prospect of mothering multiples, they somehow lose their own identity. A feeling of isolation appears to be common (Spillman 1984; Broadbent 1985b). Obviously, the more that midwifery practice can aim at fostering positive attitudes to the pregnancy, ensuring that the mother is as fit and prepared as possible for events and that family support and participation is encouraged, the greater the chance that the new babies will arrive safely and be welcomed.

■ Implications for midwifery practice

What then must be the aims of the practising midwife when caring for mothers who are expecting more than a single baby?

Research suggests that three principles are involved. These can be identified as:

- Greater awareness;
- Earlier action;
- Extra care.

■ Greater awareness

□ Awareness of parents' difficulty in asking advice

It would seem that in the past, professionals have not appreciated some of the problems and anxieties experienced by families expecting more than one baby. There was a tendency to think that parents would naturally be over-joyed. This is not necessarily the case. Mothers and fathers do not always feel confident to ask questions particularly when receiving most of their antenatal care at the hospital consultant unit. Midwives can help to overcome this difficulty. It might be possible for more 'shared care facilities' to be available for mothers expecting twins. Where this happened in Broadbent's study (1985b) the mothers seemed to establish a rapport with their 'own' doctor and midwife which overcame the communication difficulty. Perhaps those mothers who, for medical reasons, must receive antenatal care at the hospital, could also be visited regularly by their community midwife to allow for the necessary counselling and advice which they need.

☐ **Awareness of anxieties which are difficult to express and awareness of resources available**

Mothers are fearful of asking some questions. These can be anticipated by the midwife and factual answers given. It may be that a lack of knowledge made it difficult to offer such counselling in the past when little had been published on the subject. Most 'guides for parents' included perhaps one paragraph on multiple pregnancy and midwifery textbooks concentrated on the biological and physiological aspects of twinning to the relative exclusion of information about anxieties experienced by mothers and the psychological implications of multiple births. Literature is now available to assist both professionals and expectant parents.

☐ **Awareness of special groups and services**

This includes awareness of the Twins and Multiple Births Association (TAMBA), local groups which are known as Twins' Clubs, and the Multiple Births Foundation. The resources which these organisations offer to parents and professionals can be very helpful.

Midwives can introduce parents to their local Twins' Club, or to a mother of twins, to provide support. If the midwife is able to accompany a mother on her first visit, any shyness will be eased. Twins' Clubs offer leaflets and books on all aspects of expecting twins and twin parenting, provide second-hand equipment and clothing, arrange interesting talks about twins, and offer friendship from a group which truly understands the difficulties. The national organisation (TAMBA), through its specialist section known as the Health and Education Group, produces leaflets, provides visual aids, answers inquiries from parents and professionals and assists researchers with information and bibliographies which are regularly updated. Members of TAMBA Health and Education Group include professionals from various disciplines including many midwives.

Recently, TAMBA has started special Twins Clinics on a monthly basis at Queen Charlotte's Hospital, London, and in Birmingham. It is hoped that a third will shortly start in York. The clinics cater for expectant parents and grandparents and appointments can be made for any family with multiples providing their general practitioner agrees. Additional clinics are held at Queen Charlotte's for families whose multiples have special needs and for those who suffer bereavement of one or both twins at birth or lose one through 'cot death.' Even parents who have suffered early miscarriage of twins, feel their loss is underestimated by professionals, relatives and friends, and find support at this clinic. Conferences and study days are also arranged. Thus any midwife who wishes to improve her understanding of multiples or give special support to parents with particular problems, has a valuable resource at her disposal.

The recently launched Multiple Births Foundation has as its aims the professional support of families with twins and higher order births. The Foundation also offers information and advice to the caring professions, runs regular seminars and workshops on multiple pregnancy and twin problems and issues a quarterly newsletter. It provides a resource centre for researchers and initiates research ideas. It also provides a media information source. It has links with other similar organisations throughout the world particularly TAMBA.

■ Early action

□ Early action at the time of diagnosis

Immediately following the diagnosis of multiple pregnancy, the parents' most usual reaction is one of shock and disbelief. A prompt visit by the community midwife, who is likely to have met the mother already, will do much to establish rapport. Although all the questions may not emerge at this first visit, it does provide an opportunity to talk about the Twins' Club and suggest some suitable reading. This will help instil the reality of the dual pregnancy.

□ Early inclusion of the father in discussions

When two or more babies are expected the father's role is crucial. His co-operation from the earliest will do much to ease the mother's burden. The father may have questions of his own to ask and may express his concerns more easily in his own home. Fathers are often particularly concerned about the financial implications. Reassurance that it is not necessary to buy brand new equipment and that it is not practical, nor for that matter desirable, to dress twins identically may alleviate some of his worries. Fathers are also likely to be concerned at the effect on marital relations of the twin pregnancy. A sympathetic midwife can anticipate this anxiety and give reassurance that most couples, if they so wish, can continue a normal sexual relationship until the last few weeks of the pregnancy.

□ Early attention to diet and rest

It is a good thing to discuss the mother's eating habits with her at an early stage. Anaemia is more common in multiple pregnancy, but a diet high in iron and folic acid will help to minimise the supplements necessary. The midwife may arrange a visit from or to the hospital dietitian to ensure expert advice. Quality of food rather than quantity is important. Many mothers expecting more than one baby find eating difficult particularly in the last trimester of pregnancy.

Rest is vital for the well being of mother and babies. Mothers should stop work earlier than with a singleton pregnancy. Encouragement should be given to rest regularly during the day from an early stage in the pregnancy. If such a regimen is instituted, it is far less likely that hospitalisation will be necessary. The woman should be encouraged to raise her feet when sitting as the extra weight carried predisposes to swelling of the legs and varicose veins. The father's co-operation in relieving the mother of some of the household and childcare duties will help make this more realistic. Extra pillows may be necessary to ensure comfort when in bed (Bryan 1984).

☐ Early attendance at parentcraft and relaxation clinics

Mothers expecting twins should start parentcraft and relaxation classes at an earlier stage of pregnancy than those having one baby, otherwise it is likely they will not complete the course. It is also important that midwives running such classes give information relevant to these mothers particularly concerning feeding, preparation of layettes and suggested ways of 'cutting corners' (for example preparing meals in advance to put in the freezer, buying disposable napkins for at least the first few weeks and so on). It is also an opportunity to advise against dressing the babies alike or naming them similarly, pointing out the necessity to individualise them. At the relaxation class, the differences that may be expected at delivery can be explained, and the mother can be reassured that there will only be one labour.

☐ Early visits to delivery suite and neonatal unit

Parents should visit the delivery suite and be shown its equipment, earlier in the pregnancy than for singletons. A visit to the neonatal unit and an introduction to the staff and equipment will reassure her should her babies need admission there.

☐ Early detection of problems

Problems occurring during the pregnancy must be dealt with as speedily as possible. More frequent assessment is necessary than with a singleton pregnancy. Complications such as pre-eclampsia and preterm delivery are more common. Home visits can avoid the strain and expense of travelling backwards and forwards to the hospital for the mother.

■ Extra care

The midwife who is aware of the extra risks involved in a multiple pregnancy appreciates that extra care during the antenatal period and afterwards is desirable. Much of the responsibility for this extra care must rest with the mother herself and the family who surround her. The midwife's role is to educate and counsel them about their lifestyle. She can liaise with other agencies where necessary, for example to arrange home help or possibly nursery facilities for other children.

A sensitive midwife, who has the necessary knowledge and expertise, will support the family confidently and enhance the prospects for an uncomplicated pregnancy and a safe delivery of healthy and welcome babies.

■ Practice check

- Who at the moment gives the news of multiple pregnancy to mothers in your area of practice? Do you feel this is the best way to do this? What suggestions can you make that might improve the present procedure?

- Plan a suitable programme of antenatal care for a mother in her third pregnancy who is expecting triplets.

- Find out if there is a Twins' Club in your area and attend one of their meetings. What is your opinion of the resources it offers to parents? To professionals?

- If there is no Twins' Club, visit your local library and make a list of available books which you could recommend to parents expecting multiples.

- Define ways in which the father can give extra support when multiples are expected.

- What information would you give to a mother who is anxious that her twins might not survive?

- What important research do you consider remains to be done in the area of multiple pregnancy?

■ References

Alexander T P 1987 Make room for twins: 42–6. Bantam, New York

Bowlby J 1958 Nature of a child's tie to his mother. International Journal of Psychoanalysis 39: 350–73

Broadbent B A 1984 A study of the effect on the family of a multiple birth.
Unpublished PhD thesis, University of Manchester

Broadbent B A 1985a Twin trauma. Nursing Times 81 (32): 28–30

Broadbent B A 1985b Multiple births – Women's needs. Midwife, Health Visitor
and Community Nurse 21: 425–30

Bryan E M 1977 Twins are a handful. Journal of Maternal and Child
Health 348: 53

Bryan E M 1984 Twins in the family. Constable, London

Bulmer M G 1970 The frequency of twins. In Biology of twinning in man.
Clarendon Press, Oxford

Corrigan A 1977 Social aspects and psychological needs of multiple birth
families. Australian Mother of Twins Association

Edwards I 1989 Sleep patterns in twin children. Twins and Multiple Births
Association Bulletin no 28. TAMBA, Stourbridge

Eriksson A W, Fellman J 1967 Twinning in relation to the marital status of the
mother. Acta Genetica et Statistica Medica 17: 385

Goshen-Gottstein E R 1980 The mothering of twins, triplets and quadruplets.
Psychiatry 43: 189–204

Jouppila P, Kaupilla A, Koivisto M, Moilanen I, Ylikorkala O 1985 Twin
pregnancy: the role of active management during pregnancy and delivery.
Acta Obstet Gynaecol Scand 44 (supplement): 13–19

Klaus M H, Kennell J H 1976 Maternal–infant bonding: the impact of early
separation or loss on family development. Mosby, St Louis

Koo S K, Green K 1975 Twin pregnancies, influence of antenatal complications,
hospital bed-rest and misdiagnosis on prematurity and perinatal mortality.
Australian and New Zealand Journal of Obstetrics and Gynaecology
15: 179–88

McMullan P 1986a Twin pregnancy. British Journal for Nurses in Child
Health 1: 264–65

McMullen P F 1986b Northern Ireland twin study 1983. Ulster Medical
Journal 44: 131–35

National Center for Health Statistics 1978 Congenital Anomalies and Birth
Injuries Among Live Births, United States 1973–1974. National Center for
Health Statistics, US Department of Health, Education and Welfare, series 21,
no 31. DHEW Publication No (PHS) 79–1909. Hyattsville MD

Patel N, Barrie W, Campbell D, Howat R, Melrose E, Redford O, McIlwaine G,
Smalls M 1983 Scottish twin study, 1983 preliminary report. Social Paediatric
and Obstetric Research Unit, University of Glasgow

Powell T J 1981 Symptoms of atypical depression in mothers of twins.
Unpublished MSc thesis, University of Surrey

Robinson H P, Caines J S 1977 Sonar evidence of early pregnancy failure in
patients with twin conceptions. British Journal of Obstetrics and
Gynaecology 84: 22–5

Saunders M C, Dick J S, Brown I McL, McPherson K, Chalmers I 1985 The
effect of hospital admission for bed-rest on the duration of twin pregnancy: a
randomized trial. Lancet ii: 793–95

Spillman J R 1984 The role of birthweight in mother-twin relationships.
Unpublished MSc thesis, Cranfield Institute of Technology

Spillman J R 1985 'You have a little bonus my dear': the effect on mothers of the diagnosis of multiple pregnancy. The British Medical Ultrasound Bulletin 39: 6–9

Spillman J R 1986 Expecting a multiple birth: some emotional aspects. British Journal for Nurses in Child Health 1 (10): 298–99

Spillman J R 1987a Emotional aspects of experiencing a multiple birth. Midwife, Health Visitor and Community Nurse 23 (2): 54–8

Spillman J R 1987b The emotional impact of multiple pregnancy: the midwife's role in support of the family. Midwives Chronicle 58–62

Spillman J R 1987c Double exposure: coping with newborn twins at home. Midwife, Health Visitor and Community Nurse 23 (3): 92–4

Weekes A R L, Menzies D N, De Boer C H 1977 The relative efficacy of bed-rest, cervical suture and no treatment in the management of twin pregnancy. British Journal of Obstetrics and Gynaecology 84: 161–64

■ Suggested further reading

Bryan E M 1983 The nature and nurture of twins. Baillière Tindall, Eastbourne

Bryan E M 1984 Twins in the Family. Constable, London

Clegg A, Woollett A 1984 Twins from conception to five years. Century, London

Linney J 1983 Multiple births. John Wiley, Chichester

McDonald D 1983 More than one: the prenatal and postnatal care of twins and triplets. Ian Henry Publications

■ Useful addresses

The Twins and Multiple Births Association (TAMBA)
51 Thicknell Drive
Pedmore
Stourbridge
West Midlands D79 0YH

The Multiple Births Foundation
c/o Dr Elizabeth Bryan
Queen Charlotte's and Chelsea Hospital
Goldhawk Road,
LONDON W6 0XJ

The International Society for Twin Studies
The Mendel Institute
Piazza Galena 5
00161 Rome
Italy

Index